Praise for *Caring for Self & Others*

It is a healing experience to read the beautiful journey into self-caring through the wounded depth of the dark night of soul. It is through such personal sharing of self that we learn from each other. David Kopacz's book offers readers a gift of hope, courage, and self-love that both teaches and inspirits us with his soul's path into self-caring and heart healing.

JEAN WATSON, PhD, RN, AHN-BC, FAAN, LL (AAN)
Founder Watson Caring Science Institute,
Distinguished Professor/Dean Emerita, University of Colorado Denver,
College of Nursing, and author of *Caring Science as Sacred Science*

This holistic, imaginative, and soulful response to burnout is much needed in today's world.

DR. DINA GLOUBERMAN
Author of *The Joy of Burnout: How the end of the world can be a new beginning.*

As physicians, we may not always acknowledge that we each have a soul. However, we are in a sacred profession that truly holds the soul of our patients. Whatever we call it, there is a place deep within us—almost the elephant in the room—that is our compass guiding us, our North Star. Oftentimes we get lost because we don't care for our internal compass. That is the essence of what's lost in healthcare today. If we have the true soulful connection with our Self, it needs to be fed first so that we can be available to everyone else.

When we make self-care and colleague care an unapologetic and unashamed priority, we can give the best care to our patients. David Kopacz invites us to reconnect to our humanity, nurturing our hearts and minds as healers and setting the stage for our systems to heal as well.

MUKTA PANDA, MD
Author of *Resilient Threads: Weaving Joy and Meaning into Well-Being* and co-author of The Oath to Self-Care and Well-Being

Caring for Self & Others is a blueprint for authentic happiness. Dr. David Kopacz has gifted us with an insightful guide for self-care. He points to how burnout and compassion fatigue lead to losing our souls and how the loss teaches us a way into depth and spirituality. He suggests ways to sit with equanimity between the wholeness of the sacred and the mundane. This book is an invitation to show up fully and to rediscover there is no split of body/mind or between the self and the collective; it contains perennial wisdom with all its regenerative power.

MARIANELA MEDRANO, PhD
What a Word is Worth podcast, and author of
Rooting, Diosas de la yuca, and other titles

David Kopacz is versed in worldwide healing traditions where illness is approached as a loss of soul and healing involves its restoration. *Caring for Self & Others* offers a complete vision of individual, social, and earth practice where everything contributes to a communion of creation that transforms afflictions into affirmations of life. His personal "dark night" shows the way to a timeless discipline of compassionate creation with others, helping us see that we participate in a process larger than ourselves yet sustained by our unique and personal contributions.

SHAUN MCNIFF, PhD
Lesley University Professor Emeritus and author of
Art as Medicine, Art Heals, Imagination in Action, and other books.

Finally, a book that puts together what self-care and healing are really about! Kopacz, an exceptional healer, presents a comprehensive and holistic perspective on ideas and practices that can mitigate the burnout and fatigue that are rampant in healthcare. This is a handbook that will help every practitioner reclaim their role as healer and reconnect with the Soul of their practice. An exquisite, insightful and transformative work!

LUCIA THORNTON, ThD, MSN, RN
Past president, American Holistic Nurses Association,
past president, Academy of Integrative Health and Medicine, and author of
Whole Person Caring: An Interprofessional Model for Healing and Wellness

As a clinician who has experienced deep burnout, I adore this book and find it endlessly useful. Dr. Kopacz aptly offers his work as an oxygen mask. He exquisitely supports attention toward the crucial self-care healers of all kinds desperately need for thriving lives.

KATE KING, MA, LPC, ATR-BC
Author of *The Radiant Life Project*

Caring for Self & Others demands to be read with our heads and our hearts. David Kopacz challenges us to care for ourselves, others, and the systems we work in. The book is filled with exercises and meditations that can help us in this work. David also shares his journey and how he employed the ideas and exercises in his own life that reveal the depth of his commitment to caring.

JOHN (JACK) MILLER, PhD
Professor at the University of Toronto and author of *Education and the Soul*

Caring for Self & Others is a comprehensive guide that offers 31 transformative practices and meditations to nurture your body, mind, and spirit. Whether you seek to cultivate self-awareness, combat burnout, or find solace in times of suffering, this book provides a diverse range of techniques, from reflective journaling to creative expression, to support your growth journey.

Dr. David R. Kopacz's book is a beacon of hope for healthcare workers grappling with burnout and fatigue. Drawing upon his extensive medical background, Dr. Kopacz offers a refreshing perspective on addressing the challenges faced by those in the healthcare industry.

In a world still reeling from the aftershocks of the pandemic, this book serves as a guiding light for individuals seeking to rejuvenate their passion and purpose in their noble profession. Join in welcoming this invaluable resource that promises to inspire, uplift, and empower all who turn its pages.

MIDWEST BOOK REVIEW
Reviewed by Suzie Housley

Caring for Self & Others speaks directly to us in these uncertain and difficult times—a book that we must read. The author uses his own experience both as a doctor and patient to deeply delve into the different kinds of caring: for the body, for emotion, for mind, heart. It is a book full of wisdom gained by the author's insight and continuous growing curiosity about life and the importance of caring and healing. This book is written for you; that is, anyone with an interest in the world around us who knows that to live well (or thrive), we need to care for ourselves and others. David Kopacz both explains why we need to care but also gives practical ways of doing so.

JONATHAN MCFARLAND, MA
President and founder of The Doctor as a Humanist and
co-editor of *Health Humanities for Quality of Care in Times of COVID-19*

Caring for Self & Others charts a path through the inevitable downturns and struggles of our lives by using our very suffering as material for transformation and growth. It elaborates a practice of caring that leads us from our individual pain into service to others by breaking down the mental barriers that lead us to believe that there is a self separate from others. This is perennial wisdom for the soul.

STEPHEN COPE, MSW
Scholar Emeritus, Kripalu Center, and
bestselling author of *The Great Work of Your Life*

CARING *for* SELF & OTHERS

ALSO BY THE AUTHOR

Re-humanizing Medicine: A Holistic Framework for Transforming Your Self, Your Practice, and the Culture of Medicine (2014)

BOOKS BY DAVID R. KOPACZ, MD & JOSEPH RAEL (BEAUTIFUL PAINTED ARROW)

Walking the Medicine Wheel: Healing Trauma & PTSD (2016)

Becoming Medicine: Pathways of Initiation into a Living Spirituality (2020)

Becoming Who You Are: Beautiful Painted Arrow's Life & Lessons for Children Ages 10–100 (2021)

A Bowl Full of Ideas for Inventive Minds (2023)

CARING *for* SELF & OTHERS

Transforming Burnout, Compassion Fatigue, and Soul Loss

DAVID R. KOPACZ, MD

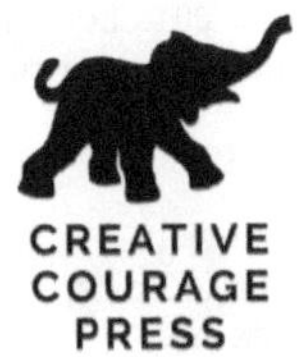

CREATIVE
COURAGE
PRESS

www.davidkopacz.com | www.beingfullyhuman.com

Creative Courage Press, LLC (Palisade, CO) www.CreativeCouragePress.com

Author's Note
The content of this book does not reflect the opinion of the Veterans Health Administration or the University of Washington and the mention of these organizations does not imply an endorsement of the book. Any mention of the author's work environment is meant to reflect upon the general health care work environment and is not meant as a criticism of any specific institution. Names and identities have been changed in regard to medical histories. Where actual names are used, permission was granted.

This book is not intended as a substitute for the medical advice of physicians. The reader should regularly consult a physician in matters relating to one's health, particularly with symptoms that may require diagnosis or medical attention. Please let yourself be cared for so that you can continue caring for others.

Publisher's Cataloging-in-Publication Data
Names: Kopacz, David R., author.
Title: Caring for self & others: transforming burnout, compassion fatigue , and soul loss / David R. Kopacz, MD.
Description: Includes bibliographical references and index. | Palisade, CO: Creative Courage Press, 2024.
Identifiers: LCCN: 2024902741 | ISBN: 9781959921028 (paperback) | 9781959921035 (ebook)
Subjects: LCSH Burn out (Psychology) | Physicians—Psychology. | Medical personnel—Mental health. | Medicine—Vocational guidance. | Medical personnel—Job stress. | BISAC MEDICAL / Physicians | SELF-HELP / Personal Growth | BODY, MIND & SPIRIT / Healing
Classification: LCC RC451.4.M44 .K67 2024 | DDC 616.9/8—dc23
LC record available at https://lccn.loc.gov/2024902741

Permissions
Rachel Naomi Remen interview by Krista Tippett, in *Becoming Wise: An Inquiry into the Mystery and Art of Living*. New York: Penguin Press, 2016, p. 24–25, granted by Penguin Random House.

Excerpt from *The Radiance Sutras* © 2014 Lorin Roche, Ph.D., used with permission from the author and the publisher, Sounds True, Inc.

Author photo: Anna Redmond
Cover art: David R. Kopacz
Interior design: Karen Polaski
Cover design: Jennifer Miles and Lisa Kerans
Editing: Shelly Francis and Rebecca Job

TABLE OF CONTENTS

TABLE OF PRACTICES

A BLESSING

from Joseph Rael (Beautiful Painted Arrow)

I would like to make a blessing to this book—that people who read it will be given special powers to help them advance their knowledge of caring for the many futures that are awaiting all of us in the future of planet Earth. For our journey has just begun and many moons and many suns from now we will travel because we are the gifted ones, us humans, we are eternal beings.

We will live forever in the Heart.

Aho.

Prologue

MY OWN DARK NIGHT

I WORK AS a psychiatrist at the Seattle Veterans Administration (VA) primary care clinic, I teach Whole Health and self-care to VA staff across the country through the national VA Office of Patient Centered Care & Cultural Transformation, and I'm an assistant professor at the University of Washington. I'm board certified as a psychiatrist as well as in integrative and holistic medicine. I have my own self-care routines, I practice yoga most days, I am certified in iRest (Integrative Restoration—a form of yoga nidra), I walk regularly, I meditate, journal, and paint—and yet I still struggle with burnout, compassion fatigue, and even what I have come to call soul loss.

There are days where I feel worn out, used up, and empty—despite being resilient and practicing and teaching self-care. In this book, I hope to show that burnout is a normal and expected part of working in health care, that we can transform the suffering of burnout through ongoing practices of *post-burnout growth.* Then we can begin the work on transforming systems that lead to burnout.

I do not want to overly dramatize or glorify my own suffering and struggles. Maybe sharing my story will help you feel less alone. It is not just you who is feeling burnout, compassion fatigue, or soul loss. It is the work we do and the systems we work in that lead to what I call the *costs of caring*—the various forms of suffering that people who care for people sometimes experience. I strongly believe that the way to deal with burnout is to share our stories and support each other.

Many health care workers have had much more harrowing experiences during the COVID-19 pandemic than I have. When COVID-19 hit in March of 2020, our team in primary care mental health integration scrambled to shift care from in-person to virtual appointments. It was a time of rapid adaptation. Like many workers who shifted to telework, we juggled multiple platforms and technologies with different secure phone and video systems. The start of an appointment might take ten minutes with signing on to and rebooting various platforms, calling different patient phone numbers, leaving messages, and waiting for call backs. Everyone was going through the sustained strain of cognitive adaptation to continually changing protocols and systems. This in itself wasn't that big of a deal, except that we were dealing with situations where peoples' mental health was often in the balance. For instance, I remember asking a patient with a bad phone connection, "I'm sorry to have to ask this again, but did you say you *are* suicidal or *are not* suicidal?"

Trying to help someone at a distance and overcoming so many obstacles to treatment and having so many ups and downs was beyond frustrating. Still, these technological and workflow adjustments were nothing compared to challenges faced by the true heroes who continued to work in person, often with inadequate PPE, in emergency departments, ICUs, and hospital wards.

Added to these struggles, a few months into 2020, a new team leader came in who worked with upper-level leadership to dismantle the team process and workflow we had spent years developing collaboratively with primary care. This team leader actually said to us in a retreat, "Leadership doesn't care if you are happy; they don't care if you leave, because we can easily replace you." Leadership just wanted us to have "fidelity" to this new model.

Things had devolved to the point that I did not feel supported by leadership. A pattern of interaction developed that when I tried to raise concerns, I was seen as disruptive. I felt very alone, isolated, a bit gaslighted even, and unwilling to open up any vulnerability to a leadership structure I did not trust for a number of reasons. I went through a series of situations in which I felt not only unrecognized for my scholarly and teaching work, but also was actively penalized for projects that didn't fit in the box. I started selectively hiding scholarly accomplishments on my annual reviews.

Working from home was a challenge for work-life balance. In fact I sometimes felt I was *homing from work*! As for many people, it was not just work that was stressful, but home and family life suffered from the constantly evolving strain as the whole world went through the pandemic. My father-in-law, Anthony Traxler, PhD, who struggled for years with progressive Parkinson's disease, went into a nursing home and died of COVID-19—around the same time I was diagnosed with melanoma. I missed his funeral in the Midwest, as well as my dad's 80th birthday party, because I had my initial meeting with my surgical oncologist in Seattle—a tough self-triage decision.

In late 2022, I was diagnosed with stage IIIa nevoid melanoma. After surgery and removal of two lymph nodes that contained cancer, I started on a year-long course of immunotherapy. I see the irony that just as I am working on a book about caring for self & others, I am hit with the marathon challenge of self-care—cancer. As a doctor *and* a patient now, my views on caring for self & other have been continually changing. I will write more about this journey later in the book.

While these are some of my personal struggles, maybe you have had some similar struggles, or maybe ones that are very different. In sharing some of my experiences, I hope to illustrate that the work we do is challenging, the systems we work in can be unsupportive, and that burnout, compassion fatigue, and soul loss are normal occurrences in this context. I am a case example of doing the right things and still burning out, still losing compassion, and still feeling like I am losing my soul in the institutional practice of medicine.

In addition to the usual stresses of working in healthcare, it feels like the United States has been growing more and more divided, day by day, in recent years. The health and well-being—the *public* health—of us all is suffering for it. This became even more evident during the

COVID-19 pandemic. Instead of working together for the health of all of us (self & other), the country turned against itself, like a political autoimmune disorder attacking the social fabric and health of the country we are all part of. There was a strong anti-public health movement, with anti-maskers and anti-vaxxers. At a time when we all needed support and healing—in a word, *caring*—it seemed that uncaring, un-compassion, and hostility were offered. Instead of caring for ourselves and others, there was a prominent "me first" movement and a lack of compassion for anyone "other," whether at home or abroad.

Just as in an autoimmune disease, people in the United States are seeing self (our own people) as "other" and attacking—verbally and physically. We are literally killing ourselves: there is a continual barrage of mass shootings with people getting shot while they are trying to learn at school, because of the color of their skin, or for as little as knocking on the wrong door or pulling into the wrong driveway. While the COVID-19 pandemic may be winding down, we live in times of pandemic uncaring. The health of the world and of everyone in it depends upon us not seeing others as "others" but rather as interconnected elements of Self, of a global ecosystem. We literally are all in this together.

Transforming burnout, compassion fatigue, and soul loss requires individual practices as well as institutional reform. A practice is anything we do on a regular basis that reminds us of what is important in our lives. In a meditation practice, when the mind wanders, we return to our breath. In a health care practice when we burn out, we can return to our practices of hope: we return to our bodies and our breath, we return to our callings, and we return to our idealism and activism to make the world a better place. In this way, we can create welcoming homes for our souls in our bodies and in our workplaces, so that we feel animated, vital, and empowered.

Working in contemporary health care, as well as in education and many businesses, can feel like you are on a plane with a big hole blown out of the side that is sucking out all of the oxygen. Remember—put your own oxygen mask on first! Take a breath. Then help others around you struggling with their own oxygen masks.

But our work doesn't end there—we need to stop the loss of oxygen by all working together to mend the hole. This hole is in the metaphorical plane we are all in, but it is also in our hearts, and in our souls, and in the black holes in our institutions that take but do not give, that continuously suck our humanity out of us. I offer you this book as an oxygen mask. Take it, put it on, care for your self—then let's get together and transform the health care system so that we can all better care for each other.

Introduction

THE COSTS OF CARING

THERE IS A story that has been told in many different times, a story that has been told in many different cultures. It is the story of the wounded healer, who grows in compassion by transforming suffering into healing. We could call this story the Healer with a Thousand Faces, just as Joseph Campbell wrote about the Hero with a Thousand Faces.

One such story is that of Chenrezig, who is also known as Avalokiteśvara, Kannon, or Guanyin. This being is sometimes male and sometimes female.

Once upon a time, Chenrezig vowed to care for the suffering of all beings. "I vow to alleviate the suffering of all beings, otherwise let me burst into a thousand pieces," he said.

When Chenrezig looked out at all the suffering in the world, he was moved to tears. A tear from his left eye and a tear from his right eye each became goddesses, who told Chenrezig he was not alone and they would help him in his quest. And then they were reabsorbed back into his being.

After countless years of selfless work, Chenrezig saw that there was still as much suffering as before he had started the work of caring, even though so many had been helped. In despair, Chenrezig shattered into a thousand pieces.

The buddha Amitābha witnessed Chenrezig's noble vow and subsequent wounding. Amitābha collected the broken pieces, refashioning Chenrezig with a thousand eyes to better see suffering and a thousand arms to better touch suffering. Amitābha asked Chenrezig to retake the vow of healing suffering, even though it is an endless task.[1,2]

In many ways, we are all like Chenrezig. While those of us who work in health care have taken a particular vow to alleviate the suffering of others, all of us as humans are called to caring in different ways. In our life's work of working with suffering, we ourselves become wounded—we lose heart, we become cynical and burn out, we lose our capacity to care, we lose the soul of caring.

I came across the story of Chenrezig when I was working on clinician wellness and self-care. This story seemed a perfect example of what happens in burnout, compassion fatigue, and what I have come to call soul loss. We vow to alleviate suffering, to educate ignorance, and to create supportive work environments—but the task is endless and overwhelming, and we end up fragmenting into a thousand pieces.

Yet the story of Chenrezig does not end in fragmentation—the healer's own suffering is seen by another healer, and Chenrezig is put back together again. This is not the kind of so-called "resilience" where Chenrezig bounces back to who he was before; rather, he is transformed to become even more capable of caring and working with suffering—with a thousand eyes to better see suffering and a thousand arms to better touch suffering. The wound of the healer becomes a gift and a blessing that allows the healer's compassion to grow. However, the healer needs to be cared for in order for this transformation to occur.

Every time I read the story of Chenrezig, I resonate with it, and it restores some hope for me. We need stories like this. For all my personal work and all my professional work, I still fall apart into a thousand pieces—sometimes it feels like on a daily or weekly basis!

THE COSTS OF CARING FOR HEALERS

When we work with others, we take on the responsibility to care. In a way, we are all activists, seeking to make the world a better place.

We strive to become better healers, better educators, better leaders—but first we must address our own suffering. We must address the *costs of caring* before we can transform from the walking wounded to becoming wounded healers. For the wounded healer, the wound has become wisdom.

Caring is the foundation of health care, leadership, education, parenting, relationships, ecology, and democracy. Caring is our human calling—it is where we are most human, most able to help those who are suffering, but in caring we are also most vulnerable. To care is to open our hearts as widely as possible. Caring is a gift that gives to both the giver and the receiver, making us all better heart-people. This allows maximum outflow of caring and compassion, but it also means that we open ourselves to feeling the pain of others and the world, and in so doing we open ourselves up to feeling our own old pains and wounds. There are times when the well runs dry, the light goes out, and caring begins to feel like a burden.

How is it that we cease to care? What is it within us that burns out? How can we cultivate our compassionate humanity and re-ignite our caring passion? Personally, burnout feels like a light or fire within me has gone out. With compassion fatigue, I feel a loss of connection to my internal resource of caring. The loss of vital energy and the ability to connect can feel like I have lost my soul, my healing power.

I have been searching for one concept that captures the range of human suffering that people feel when they are caring for others. I have come to use the phrase *costs of caring* as an over-arching term for health care worker suffering.[3,4] Here is a partial list of some of the costs of caring:

- Burnout
- Compassion Fatigue
- Vicarious Traumatization[5]
- Posttraumatic Stress[6]
- Dehumanization[7,8]
- Demoralization[9]
- The Great Resignation[10]
- Moral Distress, Moral Suffering, Moral Injury[11]

- Soul Loss
- Suicide

Throughout the book I will use the general term *costs of caring* as well as the three relatable terms: burnout, compassion fatigue, and the ancient idea of soul loss.

Burnout

Burnout has been studied across professions and around the world. In modern institutions of health care, education, and business, burnout can occur when one feels pulled in too many directions: more and more time at the computer; chasing imposed metrics, reports, and paperwork; and financial and institutional demands.

Before the COVID-19 pandemic, rates of burnout in health care workers often ranged from 30–50% in physicians,[12] nurses,[13] psychologists,[14] psychotherapists,[15] teachers,[16] people managers,[17] and senior leaders.[18] During the pandemic, burnout rates over 60% were found in health care professionals.[19]

In 1974, psychologist Herbert Freudenberger first described burnout as a term for occupational stress—a "state of mental and physical exhaustion caused by one's professional life."[20] Christina Maslach is one of the original researchers of burnout and developed the burnout triad: "overwhelming exhaustion, feelings of cynicism and detachment from the job, and a sense of ineffectiveness and lack of accomplishment."[21]

When Maslach was first hired at Stanford as a social psychologist, they didn't have lab space for her. She went out into the field and started interviewing people in high-stress fields like health care workers and first responders. When she used concepts such as "dehumanisation in self-defence" or "detached concern," she found that people could not relate to these research terms. In an interview, a lawyer who had worked in poverty law said that lawyers called it "burnout." When Maslach started using this term, people immediately related to it. This ease of relatability also caused problems, though; by using the "language of the people" it was distrusted by academic psychology and by journal editors who called it "pop psychology."[22] However, Maslach went on to become one of the best-known researchers of burnout, creating burnout theory, developing the Maslach Burnout Inventory, and spending a career caring about those who experience burnout.

The World Health Organization recognizes burnout as a global "occupational phenomenon," citing three main components to burnout (consistent with Maslach's burnout triad):

1. feelings of energy depletion or exhaustion
2. increased mental distance from one's job, or feelings of negativism or cynicism related to one's job
3. reduced professional efficacy[23]

Emotional exhaustion leaves us depleted. *Mental distancing* from work can lead to detachment, lack of human warmth, lack of caring, and even dehumanization, as we feel there is less space for us as human beings in institutional systems and that it is almost impossible to give personal care to the people whom we are processing through institutional protocols. Feeling a *reduced sense of professional efficacy* leads to losing our role and identity as a person who cares for others, instead becoming someone "just trying to do my job." This shift leads to disconnection from ourselves and disconnection from others.

Maslach and Leiter use the analogy of the canary in the coal mine for those who develop burnout. The canary gets sick from environmental exposure, not due to some inherent lack of resilience. Focusing on individual resilience tries to solve the problem of burnout by only trying to make more resilient canaries without changing a toxic work environment. This is the limitation of focusing only on self-care approaches to burnout as an individual issue. Maslach and Leiter believe that we need to focus both on the canary (building resilience through self-care) *and* detoxifying the coal mine (transforming work environments). They focus on the goodness of fit or relationship between the worker and the workplace, and identify six areas of potential mismatch related to burnout: work overload, lack of control, insufficient rewards, breakdown of community, absence of fairness, and value conflicts.[24]

Instead of viewing burnout as the problem of the individual, we should look at it as an occupational hazard. The costs of caring are the costs of doing human business. Instead of expecting individuals to build resilience in their own free time, self-care should be encouraged as ongoing CME (Continuing Medical Education)—we could even call it CHE (Continuing Human Education)! Instead of trying to prevent the unpreventable—health care worker suffering—we should focus on transforming suffering through developing supportive environments and building communities of caring.

In *Caring for Self & Others,* I will be presenting many different ideas and approaches for working with burnout. We will focus on caring for ourselves as fully human beings and developing new skills. Once we put on our own oxygen mask, we will then examine how we can care for the work ecosystem to make it more sustainable.

Compassion Fatigue

We've all had days where we felt overwhelmed and empty, like we had nothing more to give. Sometimes those days can become weeks, and months, and hopefully not years. *Compassion fatigue* is another term for health care worker suffering that overlaps with the concept of burnout and secondary traumatization. Figley, writing in 2002, stated that "Compassion fatigue is the latest in an evolving concept that is known in the field of traumatology as secondary traumatic stress. Most often this phenomenon is associated with the 'cost of caring' for others in emotional pain."[25] Historically, compassion fatigue grew out of the study of the effect of working with traumatized individuals in the caring professions. Figley defined secondary traumatic stress (including compassion fatigue) as "the natural, consequent behaviors and emotions resulting from *knowledge about* a traumatizing event experienced by a significant other. It is the stress resulting from *helping or wanting to help* a traumatized or suffering person."[26] In this way, compassion fatigue can be seen as a human reaction to wanting to help another and not being able to, much like Chenrezig's demoralization and fragmentation.

Peters' review of compassion fatigue in nursing lists six antecedents of compassion fatigue: "chronic exposure to the suffering of others, compassion, inability to maintain professional boundaries, high occupational use of self, high stress exposure, and lack of self-care measures." There are also four essential attributes: "declining empathetic ability, emotional exhaustion, diminished endurance/energy, and helplessness/hopelessness." And lastly, five consequences: "increased work errors, poor quality care, values questioning, a desire to quit the profession, and increased nursing shortage."[27] As you can see, there is significant overlap between burnout and compassion fatigue, and both have personal, professional, and institutional effects.

Some object to the idea of compassion fatigue. For instance, Dowling reviews neuroimaging studies showing that *compassion doesn't fatigue*, but rather empathy does. "Compassion does not fatigue," she argues, "it is neurologically rejuvenating!"[28] She cites research showing that empathic strain activates the amygdala's threat or pain circuit and could deplete dopamine, leading to deactivating reward circuits in the brain. Compassion activates dopamine reward systems and oxytocin, which can give a sense of pleasure, reward, and interpersonal closeness. "In contrast to empathy," writes Dowling, "compassion is characterized by feelings of warmth, concern, and care for the other, as well as a strong motivation to improve the other's well-being. Compassion goes beyond feeling with the other to feeling for the other."[29] In this sense, empathy is feeling another's pain and compassion is feeling the pain but taking action to alleviate or comfort that pain.

Physicians Trzeciak and Mazzarelli develop similar definitions of empathy and compassion.

> So neuroscience supports what is borne out through our own experience: encountering another's pain can, in fact, be painful for us, but taking action to alleviate another's suffering is a rewarding, positive experience. You can think of it like this: empathy *hurts*, but compassion *heals*. Accordingly, the key distinction here is that empathy is *feeling*; compassion is *action*.[30]

Trzeciak and Mazzarelli see a compassion crisis in contemporary health care and they reviewed the growing "compassion science" to address burnout, patient experience, and physician engagement.[31] After reviewing more than 1,000 scientific abstracts and more than 250 research studies, they concluded that "Compassionate care belongs in the domain of evidence-based medicine."[32]

While Trzeciak and Mazzarelli encourage us to lean into compassion for its protective effects with burnout, what happens when the system gets in the way of our ability to care? With all of the demands of the EMR (Electronic Medical Record system), performance measures, clinical alerts, emails, secure messages, and phone messages, the institution of health care can be an obstacle to care in the treatment relationship. It is now commonplace that health care workers don't look directly at patients—instead they type into the EMR and the computer screen intrudes as a third player in the treatment relationship. Perhaps part of what contributes to the end result of burnout, compassion fatigue, and soul loss is really EMR fatigue, documentation fatigue, and institution fatigue. All of these competing demands can push the patient into the background.[33]

The Compassion Revolution

Compassion fatigue is not just an individual issue, but rather a systemic and institutional concern. When the institution interferes with health care workers' ability to care for patients, system transformation is required. Since my first book, *Re-humanizing Medicine*, I have been calling for a *compassion revolution* in health care.[34] The compassion revolution is made up of healers, educators, and scientists calling to put the *care* back into health *care*. (I like to spell health care as two words, to remind us that we are more than an industry, we are healers practicing the tradition of caring for others).

I call for a compassion revolution because we have over-focused on technical and economic efficiency and productivity in the health care industry. A compassion revolution can be the kind of medical activism we need to treat our compassion fatigue. For our sakes as well as the sakes of patients, we need to bring back the heart and soul of caring into health care. We need to nourish ourselves as healers as well as technicians and protocol managers.

Soul Loss

Throughout history, the soul has been thought of as that which animates life. I have been increasingly using the concept of *soul loss* for the times when I feel lost, alienated, and disconnected from myself and from others.[35,36] In speaking of soul and health care, I am not introducing any particular metaphysical or religious doctrine, but rather using the concept in a metaphorical way of capturing what it is that makes us feel fully human so that we can care for the humanity of others. When I feel I have lost connection with soul, I lose the sense of being alive, vital, engaged, and full of hope. With soul loss, I feel deadened, like a thing or object in a world of objects. Maybe you have had similar feelings, whether you work in health care, education, leadership, or another field.

While it might seem archaic, imprecise, mystical, or even spiritual or religious, there is a power, meaning, and archetypal quality in viewing one of the costs of caring as soul loss. The word *soul* is not used much in contemporary medicine, although Arthur Kleinman wrote in "The Soul in Medicine" that "we need soul to specify the human quality at the heart of care in order to animate the souls of patients, family members, and clinicians."[37] Maslach and Leiter describe burnout as a form of soul loss, that burnout "represents an erosion in values, dignity, spirit, and will—an erosion of human soul."[38] Maybe what is extinguished in burnout is the light of our souls.

Contemporary educators have been warning that by neglecting the soul, we are not educating the full human being. For instance, Parker J. Palmer has called for us to "rejoin soul and role" in teaching, learning, and healing environments.[39] He also advocates for educating the heart of the student and caring for the teacher's and healer's heart.

Educator John Miller defines soul as "a deep and vital energy that gives meaning and direction to our lives."[40] Miller gives an excellent historical review of religious and philosophical conceptions of the soul. In many traditions, education was focused on the development of spiritual wisdom as well as the acquisition of intellectual knowledge. While the focus of contemporary education is largely on data and skill acquisition, classical traditions recognized the vital role of the arts and creativity in the education of the soul. Miller draws on Jungian psychotherapist Thomas Moore's work and book *The Care of the Soul*; Moore describes soul loss as:

- emptiness
- meaninglessness

- vague depression
- disillusionment
- a loss of values
- yearning for personal fulfillment
- a hunger for spirituality[41]

Many health care workers may resonate with these "symptoms" of soul loss and they can easily be seen to overlap with descriptions of burnout and compassion fatigue. But how can we reconnect to the soul when we feel its loss? In his book *Soul Therapy*, Moore tells us that soul therapy is different than "life management" (which I would say is similar to most institutional resiliency training), but rather that the soul needs daily nourishment: "friendship, creative work, community, good dining, conversation, humor, a spiritual perspective."[42] The soul needs the good life—holistic nurturing of all the inner and outer dimensions of being human. *Soul loss* provides us with a broad, general term that is evocative, descriptive, and relatable for many people. Additionally, soul loss can add a spiritual element to the discussion of the costs of caring, for those interested in doing so. Soul loss describes a state of profound alienation and disconnection from self as well as others.

Suicide

When we lose our sense of aliveness and vitality, it can be difficult to find meaning and purpose in our lives. Suicide is the ultimate cost of caring, where the clinician no longer cares for their own life. Physicians are considered an "at-risk profession," with rates of suicide higher than the general population and women being more at risk than men.[43] We lose somewhere between 100–300 physicians per year to death by suicide.[44,45] This is like losing one or more entire medical school classes per year!

We often hear a lot of statistics about suicide, but during the early days of the COVID-19 pandemic, physician suicide had a very human face: Dr. Lorna Breen.

> Lorna died by suicide on April 26, 2020. In a period of three weeks, Lorna treated confirmed COVID patients,

> contracted COVID herself, and returned to an overwhelming, relentless number of incredibly sick patients. Lorna and her colleagues worked around the clock during the peak in New York, with limited PPE, insufficient supplies, not enough oxygen, not enough beds, not enough help. They had patients dying in the waiting room and the hallways. After twelve hour shifts, Lorna would stay (as would her co-workers) because the onslaught didn't slow throughout the day or night.[46]

Dr. Breen's death brought the statistics about physician suicide and the costs of caring into sharp focus and mobilized prevention efforts. The Dr. Lorna Breen Health Care Provider Protection Act (HR 1667) was signed into law in 2023, aiming "to reduce and prevent suicide, burnout, and mental and behavioral health conditions among health care professionals."[47] The Dr. Lorna Breen Heroes Foundation website offers abundant information and resources.

Suicidal thoughts are a serious health risk and should be addressed by a professional care plan. As part of such a plan, some people may find it helpful to recontextualize thoughts of suicide as a feeling that something must change—death of an old psychological pattern rather than death of the body.[48] Jungian analyst David Rosen describes this as a shift from "suicide to egocide," in which the limited perspective of the ego symbolically dies to give birth to a greater sense of Self. "Loss of soul," writes Rosen, "and the related loss of love, faith, and hope often lead to severe depression and suicide. Regaining soul while undergoing egocide and transformation is an effective antidote to depression and suicide."[49]

Psychologist Eduardo Duran, who has worked with North American Indigenous communities for decades, also describes suicidal thoughts as reflecting the need for a symbolic death and rebirth. In working with Indigenous military veterans, Duran writes:

> Our ego-informed reality interprets the call for transformation—a process of death and rebirth—as an impulse to kill ourselves in the physical realm. The lack of a deeper understanding leads the uninformed ego to attempt its

> own demise as a way to cease existing to avoid continued suffering. By understanding the spirit of suicide and what it is bringing to us, we can have a spiritual rebirth and a completely new life.[50]

In Duran's work, the spirit of suicide could be recognized as trying to bring healing through transforming suffering into psychospiritual rebirth. While Duran is describing work with Indigenous communities, he thinks that this approach could be valid for everyone because all human beings have a spiritual dimension.

In this brief discussion of suicide, I want to reinforce that if you are having suicidal thoughts, you should get support from professionals. I also want to introduce the idea that just because you think of death, it does not have to be the physical death of your body—suicidal thoughts can be a call to transform your life rather than end it.

If you are experiencing suicidal thoughts, let the carer be the cared for—it is time to seek support from professionals. The American Suicide Foundation has a web page for health professionals, as does the American Medical Association, the American Nursing Association, and the American Academy of Family Physicians. There is also a national 988 crisis line.

TRANSFORMING SUFFERING

> If we are to transform our health care system, we must first transform ourselves.[51]
>
> LUCIA THORNTON

The health care system and contemporary society focus on restitution, trying to return a person to their previous state of health. Much of the focus on resilience is based on this principle of trying to return to the pre-burnout state. West and colleagues found that physicians are more resilient than the average population, and yet they suffer higher rates of burnout.[52] Resilience, alone, is not the answer to burnout. Maybe rather than trying to avoid suffering or rid ourselves of suffering, we need to learn to become more capable of suffering so as to grow in compassion as Chenrezig did.

As Rosen and Duran tell us, even the darkest night of the soul can be a call for transformation. Transforming suffering—rather than trying to eliminate suffering—is a primary focus of this book. Transforming suffering requires that we set aside, for the moment, the protocols of the technician, and move into the ancient mysteries of being a healer. Healing requires moving from a state of separation into a place of wholeness and interconnectedness. One of the ways we can do this is by telling stories and working with our own narratives.

Stories of transformation can guide and counsel us during difficult times. For instance, I've adapted Joseph Campbell's hero's journey model to use stories to support veterans transitioning from military to civilian culture. Through the study of the stories of many different cultures, Campbell found a common model for transforming suffering: initiation. Initiation rites mark life transitions in many cultures and provide a framework for making sense of the disorientation that occurs when one moves from one role or identity to another. For instance, the transition from being a child to an adult might involve some initiation ritual. Similarly, in stories of becoming a healer, there are often lengthy and difficult processes that include symbolic death and rebirth.

Campbell found three broad stages that occurred throughout the stories of many different cultures: *separation* from the old world or identity, *initiation* into a new identity through various struggles, and then a *return* to the old world, only now being transformed and carrying a boon or gift of wisdom found in the suffering and strife of the trials. Campbell's hero's journey illuminates a common framework found in many stories and many cultures, which is why his book first describing it was called *The Hero with a Thousand Faces*.

I've further adapted the hero's journey for veterans into a healer's journey for residents learning psychotherapy. After learning how to be medical technicians, young doctors often need to remember how to make deep human connections and attend to their own and others' stories in order to develop as healers. Listening in a fully human way is healing. Listening to and re-working your own story can help you transform burnout into compassionate wisdom.

Initiation is a model of transformation that is ancient and is found in many Indigenous traditions as well as in the wisdom stories of many religions. In *Becoming Medicine*, Southern Ute elder Joseph Rael (Beautiful Painted Arrow) and I structured our book based on the three stages of initiation: separation, initiation, and return. While Joseph Campbell came to these stages through the study of stories and cultures, Joseph Rael has lived them through various initiation ceremonies in his education at Picuris Pueblo and the Southern Ute Reservation. Since 2014, Joseph and I have been working together, focusing on different ways that people can transform their own trauma and suffering by becoming healers—that is what it means to be *becoming medicine*: becoming a healer for yourself, others, and the world.

This kind of transformation is what Lucinda Houghton and I have been working on in regard to burnout. We have been calling this *post-burnout growth*, similar to posttraumatic growth—where suffering is used for personal and professional growth.[53] Posttraumatic growth has been described as: increased appreciation for life, more meaningful interpersonal relationships, increased sense of personal strength, changed priorities, and a richer existential and spiritual life.[54] These are changes both in self as well as in relationships with others. We view post-burnout growth as not the simple resilience of returning to who we were, but actually using suffering as a tool for growing beyond who we were into who we can become.

We can view burnout, compassion fatigue, and even soul loss as calls to initiation, just as Joseph Campbell described the call to adventure in the hero's or heroine's journey.[55] The quest to reconnect with the soul is a kind of heroism that leads to healing. As storyteller Michael Meade tells us, "Life is change and the life of the soul is transformation."[56]

YOUR HEALER'S JOURNEY

The following ten chapters will take us on an inner journey—or initiation—to re-humanize ourselves so that we can regain our capacity to care. We will explore what I call the Ten Dimensions of Being Fully Human. The first nine dimensions are caring for body, emotion, mind, heart, creativity, intuition, spirit, context, and time. The tenth dimension includes leadership and caring for all. These ten dimensions build on my earlier book *Re-humanizing Medicine* as well as my own hero's and healer's journey working with Joseph Rael over the past decade.

Joseph will often start one of our frequent phone conversations by saying, "Hello David-ing, this is Joseph-ing." Like many Indigenous languages, the Tiwa language of Picuris Pueblo places more emphasis on verbs than on nouns. As I have explored this with Joseph, I have come to see that the English language's emphasis on nouns preferences a sense of separation—which can foster scientific objectivity but alienates us from ourselves and others. Verbs focus on connections between objects, which yields interpersonal subjectivity and interconnection. You can try adding more verbs in your life and see how your focus shifts from things to interconnection. You can also try thinking of yourself as a verb—a process of becoming—rather than a noun trying to maintain its objective thing-hood. The essence of car*ing* is interconnection—thus, as a tribute to Joseph I have used *-ing* words for each of the three attributes of the ten dimensions we'll explore. If you are interested in learning more about verb and noun language, you can read our discussion in *Becoming Medicine*.[57]

In *Re-humanizing Medicine*, I described the process of feeling dehumanized in medical school from the one-sided focus on objective science as the only way of working with people. I felt that I was losing my soul in becoming a doctor. Joseph might say that I was losing my sense of verb-ness and becoming an object or thing. I developed the concept of a *counter-curriculum of re-humanization* to balance out this one-sided emphasis and reclaim my subjectivity and vitality.

These counter-curriculum practices grew into the practices for the ten dimensions of caring in this book. This book is a counter-curriculum of caring, reminding us in the midst of our busy days as technicians, educators, and leaders to take the time to care. Our current curriculum and operating procedures are creating burnout, compassion fatigue, and soul loss. The proposed counter-curriculum transforms burnout, reigniting the heart of the healer, the soul of the educator, and the vision of the leader; it gives us an antidote for compassion fatigue by giving compassion to ourselves—refilling the medicine bags of our hearts; and it helps us recover and nourish our souls, revitalizing and reconnecting all the dimensions of our humanity.

Ten Dimensions of Being Fully Human

1. **Caring for Body** Your body is the foundation for your life in this world. We will explore ***embodying***, ***animating***, and ***nourishing*** as three fundamental attributes of Caring for Body.

2. **Caring for Emotion** Emotions are the fluid movements that connect bodies in the world. We will explore ***feeling***, ***connecting***, and ***flowing*** as three fundamental attributes of Caring for Emotion.

3. **Caring for Mind** The mind is filled with thoughts, invisible structures that reach forward into the future and backward into the past. We will explore ***thinking***, ***minding***, and ***evolving*** as three fundamental attributes of Caring for Mind.

4. **Caring for Heart** The heart is the place of love and connecting to others. We will explore ***compassioning***, ***loving***, and ***relating*** as three attributes of Caring for Heart.

5. **Caring for Creativity** Creativity is the place where we bring ideas into form—not just in artwork, but in the actual work of creating our lives. We will explore ***wording***, ***drawing***, and ***creating*** as three attributes of Caring for Creativity.

6. **Caring for Intuition** Intuition is a direct sense of knowing that is not intellectual or linear, it is an immediate grasping of complexity. We will explore ***dreaming***, ***visioning***, and ***receiving*** as three attributes of Caring for Intuition.

7. **Caring for Spirit** Spirit is the place where everything is meaningfully and purposefully connected. We will explore ***integrating***, ***unifying***, and ***transforming*** as three attributes of Caring for Spirit.

8. **Caring for Context** Context is more than just the backdrop of our lives; we are in a dynamic interaction between what shapes us and what we shape in our lives. We will explore ***harmonizing***, ***sustaining***, and ***communing*** as three attributes of Caring for Context.

9. **Caring for Time** We move through time and unfold and grow in our lives. We exist only in this present moment, but it is also true that we come from a place and are growing toward another place. We will explore ***growing***, ***transitioning***, and ***becoming who you are*** as three attributes of Caring for Time.

10. **Becoming Caring: Caring for All** In this final chapter, we look at ***returning*** back into day-to-day life, after going through self-transformation and initiation into ***interbeing*** (a sense of nonduality and interconnection), as we do the work of ***leading caring***—for yourself, in your work, and in institutions.

For every attribute, I will invite you into meditations and exercises, while also bringing in the work of healers, researchers, and artists. While each of the ten interconnected human dimensions we will explore in this book is a crucial part of *being fully human*, no one dimension alone captures the experience of human being. You may feel more comfortable developing a specific dimension, but ultimately, being fully human involves growing in all dimensions, even those with which you do not immediately relate. For instance, a person may say, "I am not creative, so I'll skip that dimension," but everyone is creative—it just might look different. Some people paint houses, others paint pictures, while still others paint with words or photographs. Everyone is an artist. You are an artist, a co-creator of your own life.

The ancient Greek philosophers had a term *antakolouthia*, meaning "every virtue requires other virtues to complete it."[58] "All the other virtues have similar correspondences," according to Plotinus, and "the purification of the Soul must produce all the virtues; if any are lacking, then not one of them is perfect."[59] While we can separate and study each of these human dimensions and attributes in isolation, in reality each is interconnected with the others.

After burnout, compassion fatigue, and soul loss, we can embark on a process of *antakolouthia*, reintegrating what has been separated, fragmented, and shattered. Just as with Chenrezig, we can work to gather our broken pieces in a healer's journey. That is really what this book invites you to do: to look carefully at all the various pieces of your human attributes and dimensions and start to knit them back together into a vital whole. Wholeness allows your innate caring capacity to flow again—healing yourself, healing those you work with, and healing the world.

1

CARING FOR BODY

Embodying—Animating—Nourishing

MOST EVERYONE IN health care knows how to manage a body—exercise it, put the "right" kinds of food in it, give it enough rest. Sometimes it seems in the modern world we treat our bodies as some kind of pet to be controlled rather than as our vehicle for the wondrous experience of the joy of life. In this chapter, we will focus not on how to manage the body, but rather how to live in it. Instead of looking at being managers of our bodies, we will look at how we can feel more alive in our bodies. Let's explore three attributes of Caring for Body: *embodying*, *animating*, and *nourishing*.

When you are burned out, your body can feel like one more patient that you have to manage. When we burn out, we feel like our body is an object with no fire, no inner spark—we feel depleted of energy. When we suffer compassion fatigue, our bodies can feel deadened and detached. When we feel we have lost our souls, our bodies feel empty, hollow, and lifeless. Through *embodying* we will learn how to re-inhabit our bodies; through *animating* (or re-animating) we will learn how to reignite the inner spark and reconnect to our soul; through *nourishing* we will focus on what it means to nourish our bodies from the perspective of making an attractive home for the soul.

EMBODYING

> **embody** (v.) . . . in reference to a soul or spirit, "invest with an animate form". . . from *em-* "in" + *body* (n.)[60]

> If we see our body as a thing, if we see it only as an objective biological process, we fail to understand our inward form of being embodied. We turn our somatic interior into an outside; we objectify ourselves. . . . we have destroyed the basis of our tissue consciousness.[61]
>
> STANLEY KELEMAN

The etymology of *embody* and *embodying* goes back to the roots of a *soul or spirit invested with a physical form.* If we are going to care for our bodies, not just manage them, we need to feel aliveness. We need to create a home for the soul in our bodies; we need to care for the soul of the body as well as the material of the body. We are of the Earth, through the food we eat, and we return to the Earth. The language of matter is science and the language of the soul is poetry.

The material of our bodies is composed of mostly of oxygen (65%), carbon (18%), and hydrogen (10%).[62] The soul, on the other hand, is more of an essence than a substance. Thomas Moore writes that "care of the soul" is "an application of poetics to everyday life."[63] A poetic and soulful approach to the chemical composition of the body would tell us that we are mostly made up of air and water, and so our lives are meant to flow. We are also made of carbon (graphite, like pencil "lead"), which means that we can write our own lives. Carbon becomes a diamond when compressed for a long time under stress, so we are also precious stones. This tells us that in enduring the stress of our work, we can become more precious. Carbon is also found in charcoal and soot, which reminds us that we are passing beings, made mostly of air, water, diamonds, and soot. Yet it is also said that we are made of stars—as the heavy elements of our bodies and our world came from the deaths of earlier stars going supernova.

Plato recounts Socrates saying, "the great error of our day in the treatment of the human body is that physicians first separate the soul from the body."[64] The ancients, in both the West and the East, said that we were made of the elements: air, water, fire, and earth. Long ago, medicine, philosophy, and spirituality were united. In those times it was recognized that our physical matter was animated by an embodied soul and that health was a matter of balance.

Empedocles (c. 495–435 BCE) taught we are made of four roots of air, water, earth, and fire, and that balance occurs through the action of two forces, Love and Strife, acting on these four elements.[65] Perhaps some of our problems in contemporary health care stem from a misunderstanding of how to balance love and strife. Jung describes the *quinta essentia* of the alchemists, literally the fifth essence, from which our modern word *quintessence* derives. The *quinta essentia* was thought to permeate the four elements as well as arise from them. It was at once material, spiritual, and psychological—a spark of divinity, a scintilla, found within our hearts.[66]

What causes mind and soul to separate from body? How do we end up disconnected from our bodies? Indigenous traditions tell us that a shock, trauma, or stress can cause the soul to be lost. Psychiatrist Bessel van der Kolk tells us in his book *The Body Keeps the Score* that trauma changes our relationship to our body and can even lead to "loss of self."[67] The traumas we experience are tabulated and stored within our bodies. As health care workers, we experience both direct trauma and indirect trauma, and one way of understanding the costs of caring is as a spectrum of trauma reactions. Perhaps some of the same interventions that work for treating trauma in patients might help health care workers with *embodying*.

Yoga scholar Stephen Cope speaks to the effects of a movement practice such as yoga on an individual's capacity for caring:

> As we begin to re-experience a visceral reconnection with the needs of our bodies, another amazing change emerges: there is a brand new capacity to warmly love the self. We experience a new quality of authenticity in our caring, which redirects our attention to our health,

> our diets, our energy, our time management. This enhanced care for the self arises spontaneously and naturally, not as a response to a "should." It feels naturally satisfying. We are able to experience an immediate and intrinsic pleasure in self-care.[68]

Cope's description of how yoga can help us reconnect to our bodies notes a shift from "shoulds" to an *intrinsic pleasure in self-care.* Self-care emerges from a love of Self. Our bodies naturally want to feel healthy, but we often try to control our bodies with our minds. When our minds and souls are disconnected from our bodies, we look back at our body as a thing, rather than living in our embodiment. Our philosophical, economic, and scientific worldviews reinforce a sense of our bodies as objects, separated from both the inner soul as well as the outer world of interconnection. Rather than managing the body, we can focus on *bodying* and *embodying.*

Embodying means we are not only connected to ourselves, but also to the living worldwide web of life. This is also what Joseph Rael (Beautiful Painted Arrow) teaches: we are in relationship with all life and the Earth is our mother, Mother Earth. Joseph has told me that the Tiwa language word for "self" is *nah* and the word for "land" is *nah meh neh. Nah* (self) is found in the body as well as in the land. Self is inseparable from land, and you could say that we are all living in the *self-world-place.*[69]

GROUNDING PRACTICE—COMING BACK TO THE BODY

Throughout this book we will explore different practices and exercises aimed at working with what it is to be a human being. Many people carry histories of various forms of trauma and sometimes trauma can get activated when you work with different dimensions of being human. It is not just "patients" who carry trauma; health care workers, leaders, and educators all may be carrying different forms of trauma. The idea of *trauma-sensitive* or *trauma-informed practice* is based on the understanding that anyone you are working with may be carrying trauma—including yourself. A good reference for further reading is *SAMHSA's Concept of Trauma and Guidance for a Trauma-Informed Approach.*[70]

As you use the practices and exercises in the book, remember that caring for self is always the goal. Caring for self is more important than doing every practice in the book or pushing your way through discomfort. The paradox is that growth often involves pain and working with feelings and memories you would rather forget, but if we push through pain without self-compassion, we can recreate trauma rather than healing. If you feel overwhelmed with any of the practices in the book, please take some time to pause and revisit these grounding practices. When you are ungrounded, you might feel anxious, dizzy, lightheaded, your heart might race, or you may have palpitations—basically any kind of fight, flight, or freeze response is a sign of feeling unsafe and ungrounded. These are also symptoms of soul loss, where you feel that part of you has left your body. The antidote to soul loss is bringing your energy and focus down to the soles of your feet to connect to the Earth.

When thoughts, emotions, or body sensations get overwhelming, grounding can help you find a solid base within yourself—then you can decide if you want to go back to a practice or skip it. Grounding is a way of reconnecting with the present moment, pulling yourself out of any past memories, feelings, or sensations. In the present moment you are safe, secure, and able to make caring decisions.

The practice of grounding involves feeling fully embodied. I will first give a general grounding script and then a few different grounding activities you can try. If one doesn't work for you, try others and find some that do. If you find past traumas arising that interfere with any of the practices in the book, you can seek out a mind-body practitioner or take a look at Emerson and Hopper's book, *Overcoming Trauma Through Yoga: Reclaiming Your Body.*

Find a comfortable place and posture. You might want to first try this exercise sitting in a comfortable chair with your bare feet flat on the floor. Try it with your eyes open or slightly looking down. Sometimes closing your eyes can be ungrounding for some people.

Start by taking three deep breaths, feeling more solid and present with each breath.

With the first breath, allow your lungs to fully expand and feel the sensations of your chest opening. As you let the breath out, imagine your body becoming more solid and connected to the chair and the floor.

With the second breath, breathe down into your belly and feel your hips connecting to the chair. As you breathe out, imagine sinking into the chair.

With the third breath, breathe all the way down into your feet. Allow your feet to feel heavy and solid and connected to the floor. As you breathe out, allow your body to feel solid and connected to the Earth. You can even remind yourself that your body is made of matter that came from the Earth and will return to the Earth. Many traditional cultures think of Mother Earth as the source and protector of all life.

Here are some other grounding techniques:

- Keep something solid on your desk, like a rock for a paperweight. You can hold this solid rock while you are meditating or doing a grounding exercise.

- Keep a small stone in your pocket and if you are feeling ungrounded, rub the stone with your fingers or hold it in your hand.

- Walking on the grass with bare feet can be very grounding, or any way you can gently stimulate the soles of your feet, such as pressing your feet on the floor or quietly sliding your feet back and forth on the floor or ground.

- Sit against a tree, or even hug a tree. Feel how solid the tree is and imagine the roots going down into the Earth.

You can also envision yourself as a tree, with your legs as strong roots connecting to the ground, your body as the trunk, and your head and arms as branches.

EMBODYING PRACTICE—EMBODYING SCAN

As you do this practice, let go of "managing," "improving," or "changing" yourself, and practice experiencing your body as it is in the truth of the moment. Allow yourself to notice the sensation of being embodied, of being alive. The goal is simply noticing physical sensations throughout your body. Take as much time as you would like. Maybe try for at least 10–15 minutes when you are first practicing, but later you can adapt it to briefer or longer practices.

Find some place where you can lie down quietly without being disturbed for a while.

Gently bring your focus to the top of your head. Notice any sensations. There may be nothing at all, or maybe tension, or heat or coolness. No matter what you notice, just sit with your body without trying to change or control it.

Next, bring your attention down around to the bottom edge of your hairline. Notice any sensations. If you do not notice anything, just feel what it feels like to be alive.

When you are ready, bring your attention down to your eyes . . . nose . . . lips . . . cheeks . . . chin . . . your entire face. Notice any sensations in your face.

Next, allow your attention to shift to your ears, the back of your head, and your neck. If it feels appropriate, you can let your head shift gently from side to side or back to front, just noticing any sensations without judgment or trying to change anything.

When you are ready, allow your attention to shift to your shoulders and your upper back. Let your focus drift down your right upper arm . . . your right elbow . . . your right forearm . . . into your right hand . . . the fingers on your right hand . . . and then to the tips of each finger.

After some time, you can shift your attention back up your arm . . . to your right shoulder and upper back . . . across to your left shoulder . . . into your left upper arm . . . your elbow . . . your forearm . . . your left hand . . . the fingers of your left hand . . . and to the tips of each finger. Notice any physical sensations of aliveness in your left arm . . . your right arm . . . and across your back and shoulders.

Allow your attention to shift to your upper front chest. Noticing any sensations—maybe you notice your breathing, which has been happening all this time.

Let your attention drift down into your belly, noticing any sensations there as well as the feelings of your breath. See if you can allow your breath to breathe you rather than trying to control your breath.

Notice your lower back and any sensations that arise there. Stay with your low back for a while until you feel ready to continue your journey of the body scan.

Notice the feeling of your hips on your chair or on whatever surface is supporting you. Notice any sensations in your hips. You can add some grounding here if you like, allowing your body to become solid and still and feeling the sensation of your body against whatever is supporting you.

Gently shift your attention into your right upper leg . . . down to your right knee . . . to your right shin and calf . . . your right ankle . . . your right foot . . . the toes of your right foot . . . and the tips of the toes of your right foot.

When you are ready, allow your attention to gently rise back up your right leg and into your left upper leg . . . and then gently sink into your left knee . . . your left shin and calf . . . your left ankle . . . your left foot . . . the toes of your left foot . . . and the tips of the toes of your left foot.

Pause for a moment, not doing anything at all.

Shift your focus to your entire body, noticing how different sensations can exist simultaneously in different parts of your body. Notice the sensations throughout your whole body. Spend as much time as you would like embodying. Before closing the practice, ask yourself again, what is the sensation of embodying? Is it possible for you to revisit this sensation of support from your body throughout your day?

When you are ready, shift your focus back to your breath. Observe if there is any change in your breathing now compared to when you first started. You can flex your fingers and toes, gently bringing movement back into your limbs. Allow your arms and legs to shift if they would like, and then lastly open or raise your eyes slowly.

You can adjust this practice to fit however much time you have. You can do a quick 60-second practice of head, arms, trunk, and legs. Or you can go into a detailed practice of focusing on as small of parts of your body as you wish.

The basic body scan practice generally focuses on observing and accepting whatever physical sensations are present. You can adopt the basic embodying scan to add therapeutic suggestions. If you have areas of pain or discomfort, you can imagine a color, a temperature, or guided imagery. For instance, for a hot, aching part of your body, you can imagine putting it in cool water, or a cool blue light shining on the affected part and then allowing the color to gently sink into your body. Or for a cold, tight part of your body, imagine sitting on a beach and feeling the sun, or the feeling of warmth in a hot tub.

You can vary this practice by using smaller or larger subdivisions of the body. For instance, if you don't have much time, you can group the head, neck, and shoulders; and then both arms; chest and back; abdomen; hips and pelvis; both entire legs; and then feet. Or you could subdivide into finer sections—for instance, for your face, separating out eyes, nose, ears, mouth, tongue, etc. throughout the body. Another variation that can be quite relaxing is to "breathe" into each of your joints, imagining a slight expansion and relaxation of each of the joints in your body. See if you can create more space in your mind and body for your soul to embody.

ANIMATING

Burnout, compassion fatigue, and soul loss cause us to become disconnected from our bodies, leaving us feeling empty, hollow, and lifeless. We move, but we are just going through the motions.

The word "animate" comes from the Latin roots of *animus*, meaning "rational soul, mind, life . . . consciousness . . . courage, desire;" related to *anima*, "living being, soul, mind . . . passion . . . spirit, feeling."[71] When we have lost our *anima* or *animus*, our soul, we are inanimate—deadened, dispirited, burned out, and empty hearted. Do you relate to any of these descriptions? How can we re-animate ourselves when we have lost this inner feeling of soul?

Walt Whitman wrote that he was "the poet of the Body" and "the poet of the Soul," and that he contained both the pleasures of heaven and the pains of hell.[72] The "exquisite realization of health," he wrote, was "part and poems" of Body and Soul.[73] Whitman's words were alive, animated, exuberant, and joyful.

After his experience working as a nurse in the Civil War, he continued to write about the care of the body. In an essay, "Human Magnetism as a Medical Agent," he wrote that "there is something in personal love, caresses and the magnetic flood of sympathy and friendship, that does, in its way, more good than all the medicine in the world." Whitman's view of care for the wounded was about having an embodied and animated presence. He wrote that moving through the ward as "a hearty, healthy, clean, strong, generous-souled person, man or woman, full of humanity and love, sending out invisible, constant currents thereof, does immense good to the sick and wounded."[74] Whitman teaches us of the liveliness of continually bringing body and soul together.

Cultivating a sense of pleasure within ourselves is one way of re-animating ourselves. Psychologist and yoga instructor Rachel Allyn has written *The Pleasure Is All Yours: Reclaim Your Body's Bliss and Reignite Your Passion for Life*. She teaches a shift in how we relate to our bodies through various practices, including yoga and a variant of mindfulness that she calls "bodyfulness" and "soulful reconnection."

> *The Pleasure Is All Yours* is born of my belief that disconnection from our body, our community, and one another

> keeps us from accessing kindness and experiencing healthy pleasures. This profound disconnection is at the core of our personal pain and our collective dis-ease. To embody pleasure is not frivolous; it is an essential aspect of being human. And being human means more than just going through the motions; it means feeling the full spectrum of emotions, including pleasure and intimacy in all its myriad forms. It means being present to all that is happening in the world—the suffering and the joy—and holding these contradictions within us in order to awaken our ability to care for ourselves and others.[75]

Allyn tells us that in order to be able to care, we need to overcome our disconnection of mind and body and self and others.

Moving Is Medicine

If the distinction between being animate and inanimate is movement, then to animate ourselves, we must make moving our medicine. Even if you have limited mobility due to health issues, you can still move parts of your body. You don't have to do a marathon to be a mover. Our lifestyles are sedentary: we sit at home, we sit in our cars, we sit at work, we sit in our cars again, we go home and sit at the dinner table, and then we sit in front of the TV. We have become a nation of professional sitters.

Research shows that a sedentary lifestyle leads to a shorter lifespan, which has led to the statement, "Sitting is the new smoking."[76] Here is an easy answer: take up smoking—just leave the cigarettes behind! A physician (a recovering smoker) once told me that everything about smoking was healthy, except the actual cigarettes—taking regular breaks, going outside, practicing deep inhalations and exhalations, being in solitude for a few minutes, or chatting with colleagues. All those things are healthy habits—try picking them up, just leave the cigarettes behind. Instead of a smoke break, you can take a re-animation break. Joseph Rael tells us that because we are breath, matter, and movement, our health depends upon bringing all three states into harmony—*Breath-Matter-Movement*.

What is it that animates us? Cultures around the world have words for the animating principle within living things. In some branches of Hinduism, the word *spanda* is defined as "vibration" or "divine pulsation."[77] This divine creative pulsation is an inner movement or dynamism even when we are still and at rest. Lorin Roche's *The Radiance Sutras* translates an ancient text which asks these questions:

> What is this delight-filled universe
> Into which we find ourselves born?
> What is this mysterious awareness
> Shimmering everywhere within it?
>
> What are these energies
> Undulating through our bodies
> Pulsing us into action?[78]

ANIMATING PRACTICE—FEELING VITALLY ALIVE

John Cage, a musician famous for his use of silence, once went into an anechoic chamber at Harvard University. He was surprised that he heard two different sounds after he settled into what he thought would be absolute silence in the chamber. When he asked the engineer what those two sounds were, he was told, "the high one was your nervous system in operation. And the low one was the circulation of your blood." Cage realized, "even if I remain silent, I was, under certain circumstances, musical."[79] In this practice, see how much you can become aware of the animating music of vital aliveness in your body.

You can lie on your bed or on the floor for this practice.

Go through a brief embodying scan, focusing on the sensation of vital aliveness as your attention shifts throughout your body. What is the sensation of aliveness in your head? What is the sensation of aliveness in your neck and shoulders? What is the sensation of vitality and aliveness in your arms and hands? What is the sensation of aliveness in your chest, middle, and upper back? What is the sensation of aliveness in your belly and low back? What is the sensation of aliveness in your hips? What is the sensation of vitality and aliveness in your legs and feet? Are you aware of any animating music within your body?

Rub your hands together vigorously and place them over your eyes. Notice what the warmth from the friction feels like cupped over your eyes. You can repeat this a few times, if you would like.

Rub your hands together vigorously again and place one hand on your heart and one on your belly. Surrender to your breath. Even if you cannot hear it, with your imagination, meditate on the movement within your body even when it is still: the buzzing vibration of your nervous system, your heart beating, your blood coursing through vessels, your breath entering and exiting your body as your lungs breathe in and out.

As you still your body, see if you can sense a movement, a vibration, or inner pulsation within your stillness. Invite your soul back into your body. Invite embodying. Invite yourself to become re-animated. See if you can rekindle what has burned out. Allow your breath to inspire you.

NOURISHING

Embodying and animating depend upon your ability to be nourishing toward your Self. In the United States, our culture has a strange relationship with eating, bodies, and appearance. Our materialism gives rise to both the extremes of capitalistic consumptive hedonism as well as the restrictive diet industry and Hollywood preoccupation with the ways our bodies look superficially. Add in elements of puritanical self-denial and glorification of sacrifice and restriction, and we are pulled in all directions.

We all know that good health depends upon eating a healthy diet. I don't really like the word "diet" because it has the word "die" within it. I prefer to focus on a *live-it*, a way of eating that involves savoring and nourishing yourself so that eating is a pleasure and not a sin or transgression. When I speak of nourishing here, I am not only speaking of putting nutritive substances in the body, but in nourishing the body so that it is an inviting home for the soul.

The soul loves sumptuousness, sensualness, pleasure, and an openness of living life to its fullest. Living life to its fullest also involves welcoming the "good" as well as the "bad." It involves letting the fullness of life fill us up with living vitality and passion (remember that we usually think of passion as a desire that draws us deeper into life, but the roots of the word "passion" are in suffering[80]). Invite your soul into your body through art, music, color, texture, sound, flowers, and scent. Create a nourishing ecology of the soul within your body and your body's surroundings.

Care of Self & Eudaimonia: Living the Good Life

Since the time of the ancient Greeks, philosophers have pondered what it means to live A Good Life. There was debate about whether the good life was about maximizing happiness and pleasure (*hedonia*) or living according to one's true self (*eudaimonia*).

Positive psychology has continued this age-old debate, distinguishing between a hedonistic tradition and a eudaimonic tradition in studying well-being. While some may associate the word "hedonism" with extravagant pleasure, in the field of positive psychology, the hedonistic tradition represents an emphasis on increasing positive affect and decreasing negative affect, whereas the eudaimonic tradition focuses on increasing meaning, purpose, and being true to one's self. Waterman developed a Questionnaire for Eudaimonic Well-Being that includes six philosophical/psychological dimensions: "(1) self-discovery, (2) perceived development of one's best potentials, (3) a sense of purpose and meaning in life, (4) investment of significant effort in pursuit of excellence, (5) intense involvement in activities, and (6) enjoyment of activities as personally expressive."[81] Eudaimonia can be seen as encompassing more than the presence of pleasure and the absence of pain to include a more complex perspective of knowing who one is and becoming who one is, where pain could actually support personal growth.

The word *eudaimonia* comes from *eu-* meaning "good" and *daimon*, "guardian, genius."[82] Socrates spoke of his guiding daimon. The Romans called this one's *genius*. Many cultures have the idea of guardian angels or benevolent guiding spirits. You don't have to think of your guiding spirit or "inner resource" as a spiritual entity; Jung, writing from a psychological perspective, viewed the Self as guiding the ego toward greater growth.

The eudaimonic tradition in positive psychology argues that there is more to well-being than maximizing positive affect and minimizing negative affect—finding meaning in the inevitable suffering and disappointments in life can also lead to a greater sense of purpose, fulfillment, and ultimately well-being. This distinction between a hedonistic and a eudaimonic approach to well-being applies to *Caring for Self & Others*. It captures why I am uncomfortable with the emphasis on resilience in health care workers. To focus only on "positive" emotion is not true to human experience, where our lives and work are filled with the whole range of emotions, not just the positive ones. Eudaimonia adds the dimension of meaning and purpose in the face of suffering and "negative" emotions, while also calling forth the best in us to meet the challenges of our lives and work.

Another way that the concept of eudaimonic well-being is relevant to the topics presented in this book is the idea of inner guidance. If you practice a spiritual or religious tradition, or are drawn to explore one, many traditions include the concept of a non-physical spiritual guide or teacher. These guides are described variously in different traditions as guardian angels, spirit guides, animal guides, daimons, your genius, or your soul. If you do not have a belief system that includes the possibility of spiritual guides, you can also think of these psychologically or metaphorically.

Richard Miller teaches the cultivation of the "inner resource" in iRest (Integrative Restoration). Miller leaves it open to you to imagine your inner resource in whatever way you wish, but he teaches that everyone has such a resource they can draw upon.

> You possess within yourself an *inner resource* that's designed to empower you to feel in control of and at ease with every experience you have during your life. Your inner resource is a place of refuge within you. It provides you with inner support on every step of your healing journey.[83]

The inner resource can be whatever is supportive to you. It could be a place, a person (living or deceased, whom you've met or who is an inspiration to you), a memory, an image, a symbol, a prayer. It could be a spiritual being, God, a saint, a spirit guide, or an animal guide if these are part of your belief system or practice, but it does not have to be something spiritual, mystical, or metaphysical. What I've learned in the practice of iRest is that the real inner resource is the holistic experience within my body, emotions, and thoughts that I can draw upon in my practice. I work with the embodied, lived memory of the feeling of well-being.

Call to mind a person, place, or experience and recreate it with your active imagination: embody it somatically, feel the emotions, notice how your mind responds, feel it in your heart, and allow the spirit of well-being, joy, or bliss to permeate your entire self. As you practice this you can eventually move directly to the holistic experience of inner, supportive well-being, just as with practicing breath meditation you can eventually move into a deep and open breathing pattern even while in a stressful experience.

What if we saw nourishing our bodies more as nourishing our souls rather than as gratification, appearance, or puritanical self-denial? Maybe this is the sense of balance that the ancient Greeks meant when they spoke of eudaimonia and living the good life. Maybe this is what my friend Jack Scott meant when he said, "All things in moderation, especially moderation!" Maybe the good life is not pleasure all the time, or trying to avoid pain. Maybe the good life is eudaimonic self-realization through balance. Maybe the secret of the good life is in caring for the Self, what Cope described (as I mentioned earlier) as the "capacity to warmly love the self" where we "experience an immediate and intrinsic pleasure in self-care."[84] This loving care of Self is not narcissistic, but rather caring for our bodies as precious and sacred embodiments of our souls.

NOURISHING PRACTICE—MINDFUL EATING

Mindful eating transforms the ordinary activity of eating, which is often done mindlessly, into a mindfulness practice. This practice starts even before you put food in your mouth. It is traditionally done with a raisin, but you can do this with any food. Focus on savoring and nourishing yourself.

Without realizing it, I discovered mindful eating when I was in medical school. I didn't have a lot of money and I needed to study a lot. I would buy a packet of peanut M&Ms. While I was studying, I would put an M&M in my mouth and roll it around on my tongue. The shell would gradually go from smooth to rough. Then I would take a sip of hot coffee and the shell would crack. I'd continue rolling the M&M in my mouth until the shell broke apart. Then I would gradually taste and swallow the chocolate until just the peanut was left. I would roll that around in my mouth for a while, eventually biting it in half, eating first one half and then the other half. I could make one M&M last a long time and I savored this ritual that made me look forward to studying.

Use your fingers to pick up the raisin (or M&M). Notice the feel and texture.

Bring it close to your eyes, studying it as if you had never seen a raisin before, noticing its shape and color. Consider where this raisin came from—a grape on a vine, absorbing sun, rain, and nutrients from the soil. Think of all the people who worked to bring you this raisin and all the work the Earth did to create it.

Bring it up to your nose and smell it. What does it smell like?

Place it in your mouth, but don't chew it just yet. Gently roll it on your tongue, feeling the texture and taste. Where on your tongue do you taste it?

Take one bite—just one, as you bite it in half. Do you notice any different tastes or textures?

Now you can chew it up, but see if you can chew it up completely; don't swallow it immediately, chew it up until it is just a paste.

When it is thoroughly chewed up, swallow it, and notice any residual tastes in your mouth.

What did you notice with this experience?

Slowing down the eating process creates space where you can notice the nourishment inherent in one bite of food. It would take a long time to eat a meal this way, but you could start every meal with one bite or a couple bites of mindful eating. You can even make it a communal activity with the family.

See if you can bring this perspective of nourishing and savoring into other aspects of your life: taking a drink of water, walking barefoot on the grass, getting out of bed in the morning, washing dishes, petting the dog or cat, brushing your teeth in the morning. There are thousands of activities we do each day mindlessly. If you are doing things mindlessly, you are also doing them joylessly and without bliss. When you slow down and notice the present moment, you may just find that bliss arises.

Zen monks often had long apprenticeships chopping wood and carrying water. If you cannot find bliss and enlightenment in your everyday life, it does not matter if you can attain it sitting on a cushion in a silent meditation retreat. There is a common Zen saying, "Before enlightenment, chop wood, carry water. After enlightenment, chop wood, carry water."

2

CARING FOR EMOTION

Feeling—Connecting—Flowing

> It is entirely possible to feel someone's pain, acknowledge their suffering, hold it in our hands and support them with our presence without depleting ourselves, without clouding our judgment. But only if we are honest about our feelings.[85]
>
> RANA AWDISH

EMOTIONS ARE AN ocean of feeling, an invisible internal flow that connects us—inside and outside. We will explore three fundamental attributes of Caring for Emotion: *feeling* our emotions as internal states, *connecting* to ourselves and to others, and *flowing* between different "e-motional" states.

Emotional exhaustion is part of the burnout triad described by Maslach. It is similar to compassion fatigue, with an absence of feeling and emotional deadening, like we have nothing more to give. With soul loss we feel as if we are a dead object, with no pleasure, joy, or emotion flowing through us. *Feeling-connecting-flowing* can help reignite our emotional engine, fire up our compassion, and help us feel ensouled again.

Joseph Campbell said that it is not so much that we are searching for meaning in life as that "what we're seeking is an experience of being alive, so that our life experiences on the purely physical plane will have resonances with our own innermost being and reality, so that we will actually feel the rapture of being alive."[86]

FEELING

Christina Maslach's motivation for studying burnout was initially looking "at how individuals come to understand their feelings," and "how people cope in emotionally demanding situations where they need to remain calm and detached."[87]

While our physical body feels solid, emotions are like internal ocean waves that come and go. Emotions help to get us out of our fixed and separate selves and connect us to the world around us. In *The Balance Within: The Science Connecting Health and Emotions*, Dr. Esther Sternberg describes emotions as "always with us, but constantly shifting," and that they "change the way we see the world and the way we see ourselves."[88] Emotions have their own language, which is different than that of science and disease. "Poetry and song are the language of emotions," which Sternberg contrasts to the "scientific precision, logic, and deductive reasoning" of the language of disease and science.[89]

Emotions are a different language than the language of the body. Sometimes these differences in language come out in different ways of communicating. Some people communicate through emotion: how do I *feel* about this? Jung called this person a "feeling type." Others communicate through action: what am I going to *do* about this? Jung called this a "sensation type." A "thinking type" would think, "what do I think about this?" An "intuition type" would filter experienced through a spiritual lens, perhaps saying, "what is the *meaning* of this, how does it fit in the bigger picture?" How do you tend to respond? Thinking, feeling, sensation, and intuition can be seen as different languages, and we can work to become fluent in them all. Jung's concept of individuation is the work of bringing all these languages into harmony.[90]

emotion (n.) . . . from French émotion . . . Old French *emouvoir* "stir up". . . Latin *emovere* "move out, remove, agitate," from assimilated form of *ex-* "out" + *movere* "to move"[91]

Emoting means to move, as can be seen from the above roots of the word. Emoting connects mind and body and connects self and other. At a chemical level, emotions are a flood of hormones and chemicals that give us a sense of feeling and reaction within our bodies. The function of emotions is a brief wave, giving us information about ourselves in relation to the world—and then, like a wave, receding and leaving us open to new experiences.

Feelings are what they are, but as humans we tend to classify them as "positive" or "negative." We tend to seek out more "positive" feelings (the foundation of addiction) or we can try to avoid "negative" feelings (defense mechanisms which can also fuel addictions). When feelings are overwhelming, we can be tempted to shut them off. Defense mechanisms such as intellectualization, suppression, repression, denial, splitting, and dissociation are ways that we try to dampen or isolate feelings. We can block or repress negative emotions, but blocking negative emotions also blocks positive emotions. With emotions, *to feel or not to feel*—that is the question!

We can block this language of the Self, but then we become illiterate in connecting to ourselves as well as others. A technical term for this is called *alexithymia*, the inability to have words for what one is feeling. Bessel van der Kolk describes Henry Krystal's research on Holocaust survivors:

> Krystal, himself a concentration camp survivor, found that many of his patients were professionally successful, but their intimate relationships were bleak and distant. Suppressing their feelings had made it possible to attend to the business of the world, but at a price. They learned to shut down their once overwhelming emotions, and, as a result, they no longer recognized what they were feeling. Few of them had any interest in therapy.[92]

Most of us have not faced the kind of overwhelming emotional experiences that Krystal and other concentration camp survivors did. Our defense mechanisms, however, operate on a spectrum depending on the severity and duration of the trauma. Health care professionals are exposed daily to people's suffering, illness, madness, and death. It can be overwhelming at times. While defense mechanisms can help us get through a tough time, we have to deal with them sooner or later or they will cause problems. You could think of it like having a closet and every time you find something you don't want to feel, you throw it in the closet and slam the door. Eventually, the door won't shut and then you need to continually keep pressure on it. When you fall asleep, the closet might burst open into a nightmare cascade of unfelt emotions. Or the emotional closet might get jarred open for the slightest reason. For example, getting angry parking your car in a parking lot may cause your closet to open up into a panic or rage attack.

We've all had to deal with so much during the pandemic. We have a backlog of unprocessed stress and emotions. Creating time and space to feel emotions can help us process them. The key is not to "get rid of" emotions you don't like, but to feel and experience them. You could say that *the way out is through*. If you find identifying your emotions challenging, there are a number of resources available such as Plutchik's Wheel of Emotions[93] you can find online.

Emotion researcher Paul Ekman identified seven basic universal emotions across cultures: anger, contempt, disgust, enjoyment, fear, sadness, and surprise.[94] Ekman calls these universal emotions because he found them to be present in people across cultures. Culturally, some of these emotions are considered "positive" and some "negative," but we all have these emotional capabilities within us as part of the human experience.

Can you remember times that you felt each of these emotions? If you want to do a quick feeling emotions practice, go in front of a mirror. Rather than trying to remember the emotions with your mind, see if you can play-act each emotion with your face—then once your body is mimicking that emotional state, see if you can recall a time that you experienced that emotion.

In burnout, we are not only emotionally exhausted, we are also defending against feeling, against emotions. While this choice may make us momentarily feel safer and protected, it costs us the vitality of our emotional selves. Psychiatrist Stephen Bergman, who writes under the pseudonym Samuel Shem, wrote about the defenses doctors use to avoid feeling overwhelmed during their internship year. In his book *The House of God*, the protagonist, Roy Basch, loses his larger Self in trying to save himself.[95] Late in his internship year, he describes one "side of me was filled with the horror of human misery and helplessness; the other was exhilarated, king in an erotic diseased kingdom, competent to run machines."[96] Confronted with an emotional crisis, he notices that for "a few minutes I felt as if I were on the edge of some disaster, some abyss that seemed familiar from a nightmare. Then it passed, and again I felt calm."[97] When his girlfriend, frustrated at Roy's emotional unavailability, says to him, "You're not a jerk, Roy. You're a machine," Roy responds, "A machine? So what?"[98]

Machine-like efficiency and productivity are highly valued and rewarded in health care settings. The culture of medicine and health care idealizes the unemotional practitioner who is calm, objective, does not need to eat or sleep, and is unaffected by pain and death. This amplifies the human temptation to use defense mechanisms as a circuit-breaker for overwhelming emotions. However, to deny our emotions is to deny our humanity, which dehumanizes us and then we treat others in a dehumanized way. This is the problem I address in my previous book, *Re-humanizing Medicine*:

> If it is possible to dehumanize and disconnect, it is possible to rehumanize and reconnect. That which has been split apart and broken can once again be made whole. This is a universal spiritual principle: rebirth, rejuvenation and re-humanization is possible through reconnecting with something larger than the individual ego. It is possible to re-member and re-collect full human being. This requires bringing back together that which has been separated or disconnected.[99]

The problem of emotional disconnection leading to dehumanization is not just happening in health care, but in education, leadership, and all fields that involve human beings. Is it our fault we burn out, or the institution's fault, or some combination of the two? We can keep repairing ourselves, but at some point, we also need to fix the system. We will focus on system change in chapter 10, Becoming Caring: Caring for All.

FEELING PRACTICE— DIVING INTO THE WAVES OF EMOTION

Emotions are meant to build and recede, to ebb and flow; emotional tides come in and emotional tides go out. Although we chase after some emotions and run away from others, emotions are not negative or positive—they are carriers of information about our internal climate.

Feelings and emotions come and go, passing through us, coursing through our blood and nervous system like waves in the ocean, a lake, or even a bathtub! Can you allow yourself to fully feel your emotions as they arise?

As you sit, bring your attention to any emotions arising.

Enter into the emotion. Dive into it, see how deep you can go in any given emotion.

If you feel a little sad, see what happens if you let that sadness spread through you without fighting it or trying to change it. If you feel happy, let that happiness spread through you, filling every ounce of your being. If you feel worried, let that worry spread through you, until you become worry, through and through. If you are not sure what you are feeling, choose an emotion from an emotion wheel and imagine the feeling throughout your body.

As an experiment, try allowing your emotions to flow through their natural course. See what happens when you let yourself become whatever emotion you are feeling. You may notice that things start to change in the Ocean of Emotion: one wave follows another, and they are never quite the same.

If you feel overwhelmed by emotion, try putting a hand on your heart and send yourself some compassion. You can also put a hand on your cheek or forehead. It is possible for you to comfort yourself as emotions flow. You can also review the grounding practices in chapter 1.

You can also picture emotions flowing through the larger container of your Self. While your emotions are yours, you are more than a single emotion.

As you allow yourself to feel your feelings, you may notice that emotions are like waves of information—once you experience the feeling and receive the information, the emotion will start to change, it will start to ebb and flow.

Your emotional weather can change and shift, just like the weather in the outside world. Pushing back against a storm will never succeed. Ride out the storm, appreciate its power, and maybe you'll see a rainbow on the other side.

CONNECTING

> Social relationships in organisations can be the most positive feature, while also being the greatest source of stress . . . people often say they can do the job and handle the workload, but they cannot cope with the competitiveness, politicking, put-downs, back-stabbing, gossip, unfairness and lack of recognition. We need to harness the positive power of friendship, help, humour, teaching and mentoring and consider how we can reduce the downside of social relationships at work.[100]
>
> CHRISTINA MASLACH

The language of emotions is about connecting—internally connecting mind and body, externally connecting self and others. We can feel emotions as invisible lines of force that extend outward from our bodies into the world, pulling us toward some things and pushing us away from other things. Without emotions, we are more like machines or stones than human beings, we are emotionally unaffected by the world. When we cut off internal feelings, we disconnect from ourselves and from others.

Sometimes we think that being professional means being emotionally disconnected (which is also part of Maslach's burnout triad, emotional detachment). Our belief in the value of scientific objectivity and our identity as a technician can encourage detachment. It is true, our emotions and feelings are subjective, but they are what allow for human connection. A person without emotion functions more like a machine than a human and this can be de-humanizing on both the giving and receiving end.

As Carl Buehner wrote, "They may forget what you said—but they will never forget how you made them feel."[101] How much of our professional interactions consist of not paying attention to how people are feeling and running them through rapid-fire checklists and algorithms? If we are not emotionally present and connected, it does not matter what we say if we are not attending to how we are making someone feel. Remember that Maslach tells us that emotions and burnout are intimately related:

> Emotion does not simply mark the transformation from engagement to burnout, it also mediates it. The emotional highs we experience as enjoyment, satisfaction, and pride are critical in driving important work behaviors. . . . Basically, emotions are not just private and personal, but rather social experiences, both in origin and in their effect.[102]

Disconnection is often taught, even glorified, in medicine and health care as a way to be objective and to protect against emotional "over-involvement." It is even offered as a prevention of burnout—however, emotional exhaustion and emotional distancing are also symptoms of burnout. Clinical productivity is often measured, not in terms of relationship, but through processing people as "units," as RVUs or Relative Value Units. Physician Mukta Panda has called for us to focus on a different kind of RVU—Relationship Value Units! She has been working on an initiative to create a different professional culture, incentivizing "people for building relationships and for education itself . . . giving a relationship value unit, an education value unit, and an empathy value unit the same weight as the relative value unit."[103] Ignoring the emotions of ourselves as clinicians and those of our patients does not create greater objectivity, but rather undermines the therapeutic relationship, incentivizing a productivity mindset rather than creating a culture of caring.

Emotions & Health

Being fluent in the language of emotion is necessary for our health because feeling, connecting, and flowing are fundamental aspects of health and well-being. There is an intimate web connecting thoughts, emotions, and the body. Embodiment theory studies how our thoughts, emotions, and physical postures and expressions are all interconnected. Having a certain body posture or facial expression affects the way we experience and perceive the world.[104]

One emotional state that can have a significant impact on health is loneliness. People who live alone have increased mortality rates.[105] Even living with a pet compared to living alone can decrease mortality after a heart attack.[106] In his book *Love & Survival*, Dean Ornish explores these relationships between emotions, social connection, and health. In his program designed to reverse heart disease, he includes opening the metaphorical heart as a way to heal the physical heart—meaning that for our heart to be physically healthy, we need to cultivate love and compassion. He has also shown that lifestyle changes can change your DNA and decrease cancer risks. Using only lifestyle changes of diet, activity, stress management, and social support, he showed that men had an increase of the length of their telomeres, associated with greater health and longer life.[107]

The field of psychoneuroimmunology studies the interconnection of the mind, the nervous system, and the immune system. While this is an emerging scientific field, the understanding of health and emotions is ancient. As Sternberg tells us, "More than two thousand years ago, the Greeks understood intuitively that emotions and health are one."[108] Our work and our health ask us to make ourselves more capable of experiencing the full range of emotions, for that is how we can become fully human.

Emotions as Messengers

> Your emotions and feelings are messengers that provide you with information regarding the ever-changing nature

> of reality within and around you. In and of themselves, feelings and emotions are neither good nor bad. They're neither right nor wrong. They simply provide information. Avoiding or reacting to your feelings and emotions blocks your ability to accurately respond to the world around you and within you.[109]
>
> RICHARD MILLER

In the practice of iRest, we work with the body, emotions, thoughts, and breath as pathways to working with subtle states of meditation that include joy and bliss and a sense of nonduality where observer and observed are experienced as non-separate. We will also work with opposites that arise in terms of physical sensation, emotions, or thoughts. Working with opposites means fully experiencing one state, then shifting to experience its opposite, and finally and most challengingly to experience both states at the same time. When I first started practicing this, it felt like a short-circuit of "does not compute." With time, I have been able to sometimes have a sense of expansiveness in which opposites of emotion can co-exist in my field of experience. Instead of narrowly identifying with one or the other emotion, I can experience having a field of experience in which multiple emotions arise and subside.

Another way of working with emotions in iRest is with what is called "anthropomorphizing," which means we allow the emotions to be autonomous. Instead of experiencing an emotion as "mine," we can experience an emotion as a "person" who has a different perspective than our ego. Jung said that perhaps we should not think of thoughts as "ours," but rather as a different perspective arising within us. If we apply this shift in perspective with emotions, rather than identifying with the emotion or saying, "I'm sad," we can say, "the emotion of sadness is visiting me now and I wonder what it has to say?" This allows us to have a complexity and variety of emotions.

The poet Rumi wrote of welcoming each emotion into your life as a visitor to a guest house. Each emotion can be a guide and even those that are unruly and seem destructive might be opening you up for a new experience. One of his poems, translated by Coleman Barks as "The Guest House," encourages us to view ourselves as a space that welcomes all emotions as guides that can teach us and help us to grow.[110] You can try this as a meditation practice next time you are feeling overwhelming emotions: invite them in, offer them a cup of tea, and listen to the messages they bring.

CONNECTING PRACTICE—EMOTIONS AS MESSENGERS

Is it possible for you to experience emotions as messengers who have valuable information that you need about your inner and outer worlds?

Can you welcome each and every emotion that comes to your door, inviting them in for a cup of tea and conversation? Instead of judging and managing your emotions, try greeting them as messengers bringing you important news and information from the realms of emotion.

Try doing this in your imagination.

Find a comfortable space. Ground yourself. Take a few deep breaths.

Whatever emotion is at your door, invite it in for a cup of tea.

Try asking this emotion, "Who are you? Why are you here? Do you have a message for me?"

Open your heart and your mind and listen patiently. Truly welcome the emotion at your table and allow it to stay as long as it needs. Some emotions might be quite chatty and tell you their message right away. Other emotions may need a bit of coaxing and convincing that you aren't going to toss them out into the cold and rain as soon as they give you the message. Some emotions are one-cup emotions, while some might need two, three, or four before you have heard their messages.

Before you finish, let the emotion know that you will always make time for them when they knock at your door—maybe not immediately, but that you will make time for tea when you are able.

How does this change your relationship with your emotions, to treat them as respected guests with a message for you from the beyond?

Try this practice when you find yourself struggling with an emotion, or even try practicing it once a week, to welcome in all the emotions you were too busy to greet during the week.

FLOWING

When we are in the landscape of emotion, we are flowing between inside and outside, between ourselves and others, and we are open to the flow of new experiences in the world. We can be emotional explorers, just the way some people are explorers in the physical world. To be an emotional explorer, to collect emotions, we need to be able to let go of emotions, too. Letting go means that we neither cling to positive emotions nor push away negative emotions. Instead, we ride and surf the waves of the emotional world, learning new things about ourselves and others by connecting, creating a sense of vibrant interconnection, feeling alive and filled with the sensuousness of the world. Emotions enliven the physical matter we are made of. *Feeling-connecting-flowing*—these actions create the currents that move us through the emotional world. While we can navigate these currents, we cannot control them because they are a fact of our internal and external emotional geography.

Flow

Psychologist Mihaly Csikszentmihalyi, one of the founders of positive psychology, has spent his life working on the concept of "flow." Flow states are those in which you are completely immersed in what you are doing, where there is no separation between you and the action you are doing. Sports, dance, playing music, sex, and being in nature are all states and places where flow can occur, but really it can happen anywhere. Mystical experiences are also an example of flow states where there is no separation between inner/outer or self/other. Csikszentmihalyi describes eight components of "the phenomenology of enjoyment."

1. The experience usually occurs when we confront tasks we have a chance of completing
2. We must be able to concentrate on what we are doing
3. The concentration is usually possible because the task undertaken has clear goals

4. It provides immediate feedback
5. One acts with a deep but effortless involvement that removes from awareness the worries and frustrations of everyday life
6. Enjoyable experiences allow people to exercise a sense of control over their actions
7. Concern for the self disappears, yet paradoxically the sense of self emerges stronger after the flow experience is over
8. The sense of the duration of time is altered; hours pass by in minutes, and minutes can stretch out to seem like hours

Csikszentmihalyi writes that the "combination of all these elements causes a sense of deep enjoyment that is so rewarding people feel that expending a great deal of energy is worthwhile simply to be able to feel it."[111]

Do you ever feel this flow state when you are caring for others? Healing, teaching, doing surgery or a procedure, being with another person as they go through something very intense—all of these can be places where you can feel flow states, although not if you are burned out. Burnout is the opposite of flow: you are stuck, everything is difficult, everything is a struggle, nothing is rewarding.

Follow Your Bliss

In the 1988 Bill Moyers series called *Joseph Campbell and the Power of Myth*, Campbell spoke about how to find the potential of one's life. Rather than an intellectual answer, he spoke more in terms of connecting to one's inner flow.

> "Follow your bliss." There's something inside you that knows when you're in the center, that knows when you're on the beam or off the beam. And if you get off the beam to earn money, you've lost your life. And if you stay in the center and don't get any money, you still have your bliss.[112]

The word "emotion" contains the word "motion," and thus we are back to movement again as with the physical body, but e-motions are internal movements that correspond to our outer movements in the world. What can the "e" stand for in e-motion? It could stand for *everything*, as we have emotions about everything. It could stand for *engaging*, as emotions engage us and connect us to life. It could also stand for *energy*, as emotions are an energy that flows within us and connects us in unseen ways to ourselves, people, and the world. To experience the flow of *e-motion* means we are engaging with the energy of everything.

FLOWING PRACTICE—THE OCEAN OF EMOTION & BLISS

The secret of caring for your emotions is giving them a safe place to play. We say sometimes that people who work with people should "contain" their emotions. To some extent, this is true when you are working in professional settings. When you are a doctor, a nurse, a teacher, a leader, you can't be throwing a temper tantrum—but your emotions still need to go somewhere at the end of the day. Emotions bring motion and vitality into your life.

Imagine yourself as the ocean—not just the waves of emotion, but the entire Ocean of Emotion.

Your body is the shore, and your emotions are the water of the ocean—flowing, splashing, sometimes calm, sometimes stormy. Imagine your body is like the rim of a bowl and your emotions are the flowing water that fills the bowl. You are the bowl; you are also the ocean water. Feel yourself ebb and flow, rise and fall, and then crest and trough. What emotions are flowing through you right now? Watch as they arise, build, and crest, and then flow into another emotion.

You can work with this image of yourself as an ocean or a vast bowl of water. While on break, in between seeing people, before you get out of your car in the morning, before you start your drive home, or before going to bed—practice caring for your emotions by giving them a large container to play in.

Check in with yourself. What emotions are stirring right now? Where is the point where an emotion arises? Where is the point where it ceases? Does one emotion lead into another, or is there a space between them? There is no right or wrong answer here, just observation.

Would you like to go looking for your bliss? Imagine yourself in burnout. Your ocean has evaporated, you are in a dry and desert wasteland of burnout. You know there is a hidden spring somewhere—begin to look for it. Maybe it is right below your feet, just buried. What tool do you need to find it? Imagine it in your hand and begin digging. Dig as long as you need to find it; eventually you will reach it. What happens when you do? Does the water trickle out? Does it burst up like a geyser? Imagine that this flow of your bliss will lead you where you need to go. As the water goes out into the wasteland, maybe growth starts— sprouts, flowers, and animals begin to stir. You can stay here at the center of the spring source of your bliss, or you can follow where it flows. How intriguing it is that if you follow your bliss, you may always be pushing forward into the wasteland that is longing for your bliss to bring it back to life.

3

CARING FOR MIND

Thinking—Minding—Evolving

OUR MINDS ARE streams, flowing with thoughts, like invisible structures that reach forward into the future and backward into the past. We will explore three fundamental attributes of Caring for Mind: *thinking* thoughts; *minding*—using your mind to be aware in the moment; and *evolving*—learning and creating new thought patterns for health.

THINKING

> The universe is wider than our views of it.[113]
>
> HENRY DAVID THOREAU

Thinking is a function of the mind. Thinking is what the mind does, whether you intend it to or not. The function of the lungs is to breathe, the function of the heart is to pump blood, and the function of the mind is to think thoughts.

Charles Darwin described two kinds of naturalists who used two different kinds of thinking.[114] One group he called "splitters," who saw differences between two similar animals. The other group he called "lumpers," who saw similarities. This old debate between lumpers and splitters illustrates two different ways we can use the mind for thinking. The splitter approach to the world is that of reductionistic science, which is always trying to distinguish finer and finer "splits" in the world. The lumper approach is a holistic perspective, of seeing similarities and connections rather than differences and divisions.

The distinction between reductionism and holism is a perennial philosophical debate. In medicine there is the age-old distinction between the art of medicine and the science of medicine that goes back at least to Hippocrates. It is almost like we have two different ways of thinking—one which simplifies and works through reductionism and another that works through similarities and holism.

In fact, we do have two different kinds of brains in the left and the right hemisphere, and perhaps they each have a different way of thinking: left-brain thinking and right-brain thinking. Neuroscientist and psychiatrist Iain McGilchrist summarizes his exhaustive review of the research on the differences between the left and right hemispheres of the brain:

> The world of the left hemisphere, dependent on denotative language and abstraction, yields clarity and power to manipulate things that are known, fixed, static, isolated, decontextualised, explicit, disembodied, general in nature, but ultimately lifeless. The right hemisphere, by contrast, yields a world of individual, changing, evolving, interconnected, implicit, incarnate, living beings within the context of the lived world, but in the nature of things never fully graspable, always imperfectly known—and to this world it exists in a relationship of care. The knowledge that is mediated by the left hemisphere is knowledge within a closed system. It has the advantage of perfection, but such perfection is bought ultimately at the price of emptiness, of self-reference. It can mediate knowledge only in terms of a mechanical rearrangement of other things already known. It can never really 'break out' to know anything new, because its knowledge is of its own re-presentations only. Where the thing itself is 'present' to the right hemisphere, it

> is only 're-presented' by the left hemisphere, now become an idea of a thing. Where the right hemisphere is conscious of the Other, whatever it may be, the left hemisphere's consciousness is of itself.[115]

According to McGilchrist, left-brain "thinking" is a closed system and self-referential. He describes the right brain as an open-ended system existing in a "relationship of care" with reality and others. If this is the case, in caring for self and others we may need to balance our left-brain identities as scientific technicians with right-brain activities of holistic caring. McGilchrist states this explicitly, that the "disposition of the right hemisphere, the nature of its attention to the world, is one of care, rather than control. Its will relates to a desire or longing towards something, something that lies beyond itself, towards the Other."[116]

Spiritual teacher J. Krishnamurti reached similar conclusions to McGilchrist but arrived there through meditation and observation. Krishnamurti said that thought (which we could take to mean left-brain thought) "is never new, for thought is the response of memory, experience, and knowledge."[117] Further, he says, "where the known is, love is not,"[118] bringing into question whether our drive to know, to quantify, and to categorize inhibits our abilities to love and care.

Different Ways of "Thinking"

Darwin, McGilchrist, and Krishnamurti all make the distinction that there are different kinds of "thinking." Psychiatrist Carl Jung reviewed contemporary and ancient literature on personality, as well as drew from his clinical work with patients, to develop the framework of four personality types I mentioned in chapter 2: sensation, feeling, thinking, and intuition. Each personality type interacts with inner and outer experience through a different primary lens. The first three styles mirror the framework used in this book: sensation/body, feeling/emotions, thinking/mind—and the fourth, intuition, could be seen as comprising intuition and spiritual dimensions. Jung believed that everyone had a primary and secondary "personality type," and that the other modes were relatively undeveloped and unconscious.

The implications of this theory are that people process experiences in different ways: sensation types process through their bodies, feeling types process through their emotions, thinking types process through their minds, while intuitive types process through intuition and spiritual domains. We could say that people "think" in different ways—some *think* with their bodies first, others with their emotions, some with their minds, and others from a spiritual perspective.

Jung's theory of personal growth, which he called individuation, was dynamic. While we might start off with a particular form of processing being our "comfort zone," as we grow, life challenges us to grow in the functions we are not as comfortable with. His concept of the crisis of mid-life often corresponded to a need to shift one's primary mode of approaching and processing experiences. If one started off as a thinking type, the challenge in later life would be to develop awareness of bodily sensation. We all use all four of the different functions of sensation, feeling, thinking, and intuition, but Jung taught that we each have a personality type that tends to favor some of these functions over others.

Social psychology supports the idea that what we focus on can blind us to other aspects of reality. For instance, we might think that we can multi-task and pay attention to more than one thing at a time, but research contradicts this belief. Classic studies by Chabris and Simons showed that if subjects were involved in an attention task, such as counting how many passes a basketball team makes, that 50% of the time they would not see someone in a gorilla suit walk on to the court![119] This study has implications for health care as our default is to be multi-tasking: listening to a patient, looking up labs, reading the electronic medical record, maybe even typing a note while interviewing the patient, and also attending to a series of beeps and alerts from pages, cell phones, instant message systems, emails, overhead hospital alerts, and wall phones. Other authors have done a follow-up study placing an image of a gorilla (48 times the size of a typical lung nodule) in chest CT scans and found that 83% of radiologists did not see the unexpected finding.[120] This phenomenon is called "sustained inattentional blindness." We tend to see what we expect to see and overlook what we do not expect to see.

Our minds influence our perceptions, which creates our reality. Buddhist nun Pema Chödrön gives an example of how we mentally create our own realities. She tells of a samurai who confronts a wise man and wants to be taught the nature of heaven and hell. The wise man proceeds to insult the samurai, who grows more and more angry and threatens to cut off his head. The wise man calmly says, "That's hell." The samurai starts to cry and begs forgiveness of the teacher, who then says, "That's heaven." Chödrön summarizes, "There isn't any hell or heaven except for how we relate to our world."[121]

THINKING PRACTICE—MAPPING YOUR LIFE

Thinking is a way to structure your life in a linear way. Thinking is generally about reflecting on the past or planning for the future and this can be a helpful skill in mapping your life. You can use your thinking capacity to plan out your life. In this practice, focus on the next year of your life.

In your journal or with some blank pieces of paper, write out the names of the coming months.

Take a deep breath, connect to your body, and connect to your emotions. Now activate your thinking mind and think about your dreams and goals for the coming month. Write down what comes to you.

Let your mind wander. The sky is the limit for your dreams, or maybe even the stars! Repeat this process for each month. Don't worry about planning out the details—that is the next part of the exercise and you will come back to it later. Let yourself build castles in the sky!

> I learned this at least, by my experiment; that if one advances confidently in the direction of his dreams, and endeavors to live the life which he has imagined, he will meet with success unexpected in common hours . . . If you have built castles in the air, your work need not be lost; that is where they should be. Now put foundations under them.[122]
>
> HENRY DAVID THOREAU

Once you have filled in each of the twelve months, go back and write out some bullet points of what you would need to do to reach these goals. This is where thinking comes in, by helping you bring your dreams down to earth and to operationalize and realize them. For instance, if you want to get back to painting, or learn to paint, your goals might be things like: buy some paint and materials; look into what classes are available in the community or at colleges and universities or look online for what you can learn for free; set aside a certain amount of time each week or month to paint; spend some time getting inspiration from nature or looking at other artists' work. You can have as many goals as you want—just be realistic as to what you can accomplish and then think out what steps you need to take to accomplish each goal.

After you've done this for twelve months, you can do some future planning if you would like. Dedicate a page for the next year, a page for the next five years, and a page for the next ten years. What are your longer-term goals? Do you want to become certified as a yoga instructor? Do you want to travel somewhere? Do you want to take some classes or get a degree or learn a language or skill? For each page, take a few deep breaths, and then see what arises.

Now this is where thinking comes in again. You've envisioned different dreams for your life, but now narrow it down and make it more linear using thinking. What are the next practical steps you need to take to move toward your goals?

The function of thinking (left brain) can help you take the big dreams and break them down into smaller, achievable steps. Breaking your life down into segments can make life seem more manageable and can also help you remember and reconnect to what is important in your life. Thinking can help build the steps or the bridge to achieve your dreams, connecting where you are now to your castles in the air. For dreams and inspirations, though, you may need right-brain thinking.

MINDING

> Mindfulness is awareness, cultivated by paying attention in a sustained and particular way: on purpose, in the present moment, and nonjudgmentally. It is one of the many forms of meditation, if you think of meditation as any way in which we engage in 1) systematically regulating our attention and energy, 2) thereby influencing and possibly transforming the quality of our experience, 3) in the service of realizing the full range of our humanity, and of 4) our relationship to others and the world.[123]
>
> JON KABAT-ZINN

This description of mindfulness is in distinction from our common mode of thinking. Whereas thinking is often about remembering the past or planning for the future, Kabat-Zinn tells us that mindfulness is about being in the present moment. Mindfulness is a field and practice that has been growing in popularity for working with personal growth and stress reduction, as well as for physical and mental health and well-being. While the word "mind" is in mindfulness, this is more than just a mental practice, as it entails allowing the language of the mind to speak without only listening to that language. Mindfulness can lead to enhanced embodiment as well as to a greater sense of emotional well-being by allowing the body and emotions to speak as well as the mind.

Interestingly, McGilchrist points out that studies of mindfulness meditation, shamanic states, and many religious states show greater right-brain hemisphere activation. This contrasts the kind of thinking or observation in mindfulness (right brain) with what we generally consider when we think of thinking (left brain). "Spiritual practices," writes McGilchrist, "such as meditation are designed purposely to transcend typical left hemisphere reactions to perceived events."[124]

Wolf and Serpa, in their book *A Clinician's Guide to Teaching Mindfulness*, describe four different foundations of mindfulness:

1. Mindfulness of the body
2. Mindfulness of feeling tones

3. Mindfulness of the mind
4. Mindfulness of how the mind operates[125]

Mindfulness can look back to observe emotions, the body—it can even observe itself, and its own inner operations. Without developing some degree of minding, you are letting your thoughts, emotions, and body run amuck—as no one is minding the shop, no one is minding your business!

While there is often a Buddhist undercurrent to mindfulness, it is applicable for anyone, regardless of their worldview or religion. Psychologist Christopher Germer has worked on adapting mindfulness into psychotherapy. He summarizes the Buddha's Four Noble Truths:

1. The human condition involves suffering.
2. The conflict between how things are and how we desire them to be causes this suffering.
3. Suffering can be reduced or eliminated by changing our attitude toward unpleasant experience.
4. There are eight general strategies (the Eightfold Path) to bring suffering to an end.[126]

The Buddha's teachings are very similar to the work of psychotherapy: the alleviation of human suffering. However, as the Four Noble Truths show, suffering is inherent in life and the way to work with it is to change our attitude toward suffering, rather than to eliminate it.

Mindfulness is a technical term as well as a concept that is used generally in popular culture. Without getting into the technical mindfulness terminology, I will use the verb, *minding*, as a function of the mind being mindful. Minding is a process of identifying with a larger Self rather than with each passing thought, emotion, or sensation. It is also a quality of presence. Minding entails a kind of stewardship of our thoughts, emotions, and physical sensations—we watch them, making sure they don't get into too much trouble, but we don't follow them around in circles or follow them over the cliff.

Most people, when they sit down to practice minding, say that they can't do it because their mind is too busy—because they identify with their thoughts. The mind's job is to think; the Self's job is to take in what the mind says as one of many different languages and dimensions of the Self. Minding is not controlling or stopping one's thoughts, it is to allow one's thoughts to peacefully co-exist with one's body and emotions. We see that there is more to us than our bodies, our emotions, and our thoughts.

While we might think of Pandora's box from Greek mythology as a story that tells us we need to lock away everything negative and never open the box, the word *pan-dora* means *all-giving*. Many things viewed from the limited perspective of the ego seem like calamities, but when viewed from the perspective of the Self, these negative things are gifts that help us grow beyond the limitations of who we once were. In the movie *Jacob's Ladder*, the angel-like chiropractor Louie quotes the medieval writer Meister Eckhart,

> Eckhart saw Hell too. He said: The only thing that burns in Hell is the part of you that won't let go of life, your memories, your attachments. They burn them all away. But they're not punishing you, he said. They're freeing your soul. So, if you're frightened of dying and . . . you're holding on, you'll see devils tearing your life away. But if you've made your peace, then the devils are really angels, freeing you from the earth.[127]

It can feel like hell, sitting with your thoughts, emotions, and sensations—but these are all you, and by minding them in the moment, they become healing.

Minding for Meaning & Happiness

> When we are no longer able to change a situation . . . we are challenged to change ourselves.[128]
>
> VIKTOR FRANKL

While a Buddhist perspective would teach us that the flow of our thoughts follows attachments to pleasure and tries to avoid experiences of pain, we can also see that there is an inherent search for meaning that occurs within our minds. Meaning is a higher-level function that fits together the pieces of our body, emotions, and thoughts.

Viktor Frankl, a Holocaust survivor and psychiatrist, focused on how we create meaning and how we shape our experience of the world based on our thoughts. He wrote *Man's Search for Meaning*, where he developed the idea of logotherapy (meaning centered psychotherapy) and he was influential in the philosophy of existentialism. Frankl wrote that "everything can be taken from a man but one thing: the last of human freedoms—to choose one's attitude in any given set of circumstances, to choose one's own way."[129]

Frankl realized that happiness cannot be a goal in and of itself, rather it is a by-product of reason and meaning in life:

> But happiness cannot be pursued; it must ensue. One must have a reason to "be happy." Once the reason is found, however, one becomes happy automatically. As we see, a human being is not one in pursuit of happiness but rather in search of a reason to become happy, last but not least, through actualizing the potential meaning inherent and dormant in a given situation.[130]

For Frankl, happiness is a product of meaning. However, both meaning and happiness can be elusive; the more we grasp after them, the more they recede. While it may seem we can create meaning through the power of our mind and thoughts, happiness seems more like something that happens when our mind gets out of the way. While the field of cognitive behavioral therapy looks at the way we create our unhappiness through having negative or unrealistic expectations (not unlike with Buddhism), there is also the aforementioned field of positive psychology—how our thoughts can create well-being. For so long we have studied disease and the pathologies of why we are sick. Positive psychology turns its focus on how we can be healthy and have well-being. Rather than viewing health as the absence of disease, we can start to turn to ways that we can create happiness in our lives.

In *Hector and the Search for Happiness* (a book that has also been made into a movie by the same name), author and psychiatrist

François Lelord explores some of these issues. Hector is a psychiatrist who realizes that even though his private clients seem to have everything, they are unhappy about the smallest things. Hector sets off on a trip around the world to research what happiness is. At first, he thinks he is doing this for his patients, but he soon realizes he is doing it for himself. In the book, he comes up with twenty-three rules of happiness. Here are a few:

1. Happiness often comes when least expected
2. Happiness is a long walk in beautiful, unfamiliar mountains
3. It's a mistake to think that happiness is the goal
4. Happiness is being with the people you love; unhappiness is being separated from the people you love
5. Happiness is doing a job you love
6. Happiness is feeling useful to others
7. Happiness comes when you feel truly alive
8. Happiness is a certain way of seeing things
9. Happiness means making sure that those around you are happy[131]

Hector's rules of happiness are akin to the findings of positive psychology. Through minding, we can cultivate a practice of gratitude and happiness.

While we are focusing on mindfulness and minding in this chapter, mindfulness may start with the mind, but it leads to the heart, which is our next chapter. As Jon Kabat-Zinn tells us, mindfulness is as much about the heart as it is about the mind.

> Moreover, when we speak of *mindfulness*, it is important to keep in mind that we equally mean *heartfulness*. In fact, in Asian languages, the word for "mind" and the word for "heart" are usually the same. So if you're not hearing or feeling the word *heartfulness* when you encounter or use the word *mindfulness*, you are in all likelihood missing its essence.[132]

MINDING PRACTICE—PRACTICING MINDFULNESS

Minding is a state of self-observation and acceptance of the present moment—which can lead to experiences of meaning and well-being. Minding develops the capacity to be aware of and observe your physical sensations, your emotions, and your thoughts—all the while recognizing that you are more than your sensations, feelings, and thoughts.

The Self is an observer of these passing states. Most of us identify with our sensations, feelings, and thoughts and react to them immediately. Through minding, however, you can notice that you are having sensations, emotions, and thoughts and realize that they are occurring within you, but that your awareness is larger than what passes through. Sensations, emotions, and thoughts are like fish in a stream, or leaves floating on water, or like waves in the ocean—they are human phenomena occurring within the Self.

The following practice has two parts. The first is to watch your thinking. The second is to use minding to watch your thoughts without identifying with them.

Step I: Thinking

Take a few deep breaths. Let yourself go in the flow of your thoughts. It might seem like this:

"I'm uncomfortable/I have an itch/this is dumb/I don't think I'm doing it right/I'm dumb/gosh I'm kind of sad—I wonder why/oh I can't believe what that person said to me—how mean they are/I'm hungry, I wonder what I'll have for lunch/that driver this morning really pissed me off, what a jerk!/I'm really angry now/I am so angry/I'm still angry/darn, I'm clenching my teeth/is it time to go to the dentist/I'm afraid of the dentist/I don't think I'll go/I should go/I don't want to/I should go though/I wonder what I'd look like with no teeth?/ok, I'll go to the dentist/my foot is numb/oh yeah, I'm supposed to breathe/ok, I took a breath/now what?/ok, I'll take another breath/oh yeah..."

Everyone's mind is like this. Many people say that they cannot meditate because their minds are too busy—that's just what it is to have a human mind, it is always busy. Your mind's job is to think. Your Self's job is to direct the mind to think about the tasks you want to accomplish and not let your mind take over as boss of you. The first stage of minding is to be aware of what your mind is doing, not necessarily changing it. It is like minding a shop—you never know who will be the next customer!

Here is teacher Ramana Maharshi's advice on meditation:

> Do not meditate—be!
> Do not think you are—be!
> Don't think about being—you are![133]

Step II: Minding

If you would like to practice minding, find a comfortable meditation posture. Sometimes this is called a noble posture—feet on the floor if you are sitting in a chair, or creating a stable base if you are sitting on the floor; spine tall but not stiff, neck and head reaching toward the sky, but not straining. Actually, just getting into a comfortable and alert posture is, itself, a form of minding.

Take a few deep breaths. Pace your breathing so it is deep and steady. If you get lost in your thoughts, come back to your breath. Or you can follow Ramana Maharshi's advice: be, don't think about being.

Allow your field of consciousness to expand. See if you can allow your consciousness to expand a little beyond the confines of your skin to feel the room around you. Allow a sense of inner openness. See if you can imagine yourself as a hollow bone or hollow tube. Practice meeting your thinking with opening. Welcome everything: thoughts, emotions, sensations—everything, but at the same time remember that you are also more than your momentary thoughts, emotions, and sensations.

In the beginning, try doing this for five minutes. You can set a timer if you like. As you feel comfortable, try extending the time, working up to ten minutes, then fifteen minutes.

Minding is a practice, just as living is a practice. It is not about being perfect or making your physical sensations, emotions, and thinking do what you want them to do. It is more like becoming comfortable in the ecosystem of your body, emotions, and mind.

EVOLVING

> There is no single word for meditation in the original language of Buddhism. The closest is one that translates as "mental development."[134]
>
> MARK EPSTEIN

Learning occurs when you have an open mind. Being open to learning is how we grow and evolve and move from who we were to who we are becoming. To evolve, we have to be open to change. It is a strange paradox that we must accept what we wish to change in order to change it. Acceptance opens the mind so that it can change. You are not just changing a momentary thought, but you are changing your deep personality. In other words, you are not just changing a thought, you are changing the structure of yourself that gives rise to thoughts.

> **evolve** (v.) "to unfold, open out, expand," from Latin *evolvere* "to unroll, roll out, roll forth, unfold," especially of books; figuratively "to make clear, disclose; to produce, develop,". . . from PIE [Proto-Indo-European] root **wel-* (3) "to turn, revolve." Meaning "to develop by natural processes to a higher state"[135]

The etymology of *evolving* does not necessarily have the implication of linear progress that we often think of with evolution. *Unrolling, unfolding* like a book, *making clear, disclosing*, and *to turn* or *revolve*—all these meanings of evolving remind us of Jung's circumambulation of the Self, the perpetual unfolding of individuation and becoming who you are. Darwin only used the word "evolution" once in *On the Origin of Species*; instead he preferred "descent with modification."[136] Descent with modification sounds like the first part of initiation: descending into the abyss, the dark night of the soul, or maybe even burnout or compassion fatigue or soul loss. The transformational modification experienced in the depths is what allows for the ascending journey, the return. In evolving, we do not so much leave something behind as expand, much like Chenrezig after exploding into a thousand pieces evolved a thousand arms and eyes to better touch and see suffering.

Philosopher Ken Wilber described that "evolution is a process of transcend and include," in which "the wholeness *transcends* but the parts are *included*."[137] This is a holistic expansion, a spherical growth rather than linear growth. In fact, aren't our lives this way? Earlier events and experiences in our lives remain, even though we grow and evolve as we take the road less traveled in life.

> [E]volution is best thought of as *Spirit-in-action*, God-in-the-making, where Spirit unfolds itself at every stage of development, thus manifesting more of itself, and realizing more of itself, at every unfolding. Spirit is not some particular stage . . . but rather the entire process of unfolding itself, an infinite process that is completely present at every finite stage, but becomes more available to itself with every evolutionary opening.[138]

Evolving is a process of unfolding, uncovering, and discovering. Rather than competition for the "survival of the fittest," we in health care are striving to create an environment that promotes caring for the survival of all. We are evolving from the narrow boundaries of ego to expand outward to *care for self & others.*

Quantum physicist David Bohm describes nature and evolution as "a *creative process,* in which not merely new structures, but also new orders of structure are always emerging."[139] He sees an "organizing energy"[140] at work that is always creating more complex, interrelated structures. The evolving we are trying to do in health care is around caring, creating an organizing structure of care within which we can do our caring work. Caring is based on intimate relationship and closeness in which we do not see the other as alien, but rather as like us or even part of us. To care for others is to see the Self in others.

We are trying to evolve hospitals and clinics as Houses of Care, rather than Houses of Billing Codes and Procedures. Bohm describes the root of the word "economy" relating back to the Greek "household management."

> The earth is one household really, but we are not treating it that way. So the first step in economics is to say: "The earth is one household. It is all one." . . To see that everybody not merely *depends* on everybody, but actually is everybody in a deeper sense. We are the earth, because all our substance comes from the earth and goes back to it. It is a mistake to say it is an environment just surrounding us, because that would be like the brain regarding the rest of the body as part of its environment. It is essential to see the world as one, because these households are not independent.[141]

Bohm's nondual perspective encourages our minds to evolve beyond ourselves as separate beings, to see that we are all one household, we are each only a part of a larger whole. When our minds can evolve this way, *caring for self & others* is a natural unfolding of our identity as *all one.*

EVOLVING PRACTICE—EVOLVING BEYOND EGO

Thinking is a relatively narrow function of the mind. Thinking separates one thing from another, one moment from another, making categories and divisions. Minding is a more open and inclusive function of the mind, which has the capacity for observation. Evolving is the capacity of the mind to grow beyond itself, beyond old forms and identities. In caring for self & others, we think of the ego as being comprised of the body, emotions, and mind. One of the functions of the mind is to be able to evolve beyond itself. Rather than seeing the ego as the pinnacle of evolution, it is possible to see the mind as possessing the capacity to evolve beyond ego to love. Whereas the ego is focused on the small self of body-emotion-mind, love is a function of the heart and is inclusive rather than exclusive. This does not mean that the ego is "bad," just limited compared to our potential experience of evolving beyond our self-imposed limitations.

Begin by finding a comfortable posture.

Take a few deep breaths.

Notice your body. Notice any physical sensations you might be having.

Next, notice your emotions. Feel the ebb and flow of emotions arising within you.

When you are ready, allow your focus to shift to your thoughts, with thinking flowing through your mind.

Allow yourself to experience your ego: the integration of body, emotions, and mind. Notice yourself as a distinct and discrete unit from those around you and from your environment. Notice the possessive feeling of the ego: my body, my emotions, my thoughts.

When you are ready, allow the evolving function of the mind to begin to transcend itself. Maybe this happens automatically, but it can be a challenging shift to make. You can imagine your awareness extending beyond your skin; allow the evolving function of the mind to expand to fill the whole room. Allow this shift from "me" to an interconnected network. See if you can experience, even for a moment, a sense of interconnectedness between you and everything in the room. This is a figure/ground shift.

Here is another practice.

The oxygen that you breathe comes from plants. The carbon dioxide you exhale is "breathed" in by plants and turned back into oxygen. In your imagination, trace the oxygen and carbon dioxide back and forth between yourself and a plant or tree. It can be a plant in your home, or a tree on the street—whatever green being that presents itself to your imagination is perfect.

> Follow the flow of carbon dioxide out of your lungs as it's taken in by the chlorophyll of your green breathing partner and transformed from carbon dioxide back into oxygen, and then breathe that into your lungs. Follow this loop for as many cycles as you would like.

To situate the ego within the larger context of life can occur through the evolving function of the mind. Children are more evolved than adults in some ways because this interconnection is natural to them. As we become more involved with our egos, we can actually become less evolved—but the mind has the solution to this problem that the separation of thinking can create.

Next, let us evolve from the ego to the heart. Remember that Ken Wilber describes this kind of evolution as *transcending and including*. The goal is not to negate the ego, but to situate the ego in its proper relationship with others and the world.

4

CARING FOR HEART

Compassioning—Loving—Relating

The heart is a pump that needs to be addressed on a physical level, but our hearts are more than just pumps. A true physician is more than just a plumber, technician, or mechanic. We also have an emotional heart, a psychological heart, and a spiritual heart.[142]

DEAN ORNISH

The sole purpose of life is to grow. The ultimate lesson is learning how to love and be loved unconditionally. . . . All the hardships that come to you in life, all the tribulations and nightmares, all the things you see as punishments from God, are in reality like gifts. They are an opportunity to grow, which is the sole purpose of life. You cannot heal the world without healing yourself first. . . . Everything is bearable when there is love. My wish is that you try to give more people more love. The only thing that lives forever is love.[143]

ELISABETH KÜBLER-ROSS

THE HEART IS the place of love, where our boundaries and identities open beyond our egos. We will explore three fundamental attributes of Caring for Heart—*compassioning* (feeling with others), *loving* (opening our hearts), and *relating* (connecting through compassioning and loving to others and the world).

The body, emotions, and mind are self-centered; the heart is other-centered. Humanitarian work, sacrifice, and putting others first all come from the heart. While a technician only needs the mind, the heart is necessary to become a healer. Thus, burnout extinguishes the flame of the healer's heart. Compassion fatigue exhausts our ability to care for others. Soul loss leaves our hearts empty and vacant, alone in the world even when we are surrounded by others. Caring for the heart helps us to reignite the heart and soul of the healer and to refill the medicine bags of our hearts with compassion for self & others.

COMPASSION-ING

> **compassion** (n.) . . . from Old French *compassion* "sympathy, pity". . . Late Latin *compassionem* . . . "sympathy,". . . *compati* "to feel pity," from *com-* "with, together" + *pati* "to suffer"[144]

Compassion literally means *to feel or suffer with*. Much of our technical training teaches us to be objective, which is the opposite of *feeling with*. There is so much stress and time-pressure in the hospital and clinic setting that most staff don't feel they have time *to feel*, even if they can get past their objectivity. This leads to the uncaring, disconnected assembly line provision of techniques. What do you think happens to "health care" if we lose the *care*? Even the word "health" leads us back to wholeness and healing.

> **health** (n.) Old English *hælþ* "wholeness, a being whole, sound or well," from Proto-Germanic **hailitho*, from PIE **kailo-* "whole, uninjured, of good omen" (source also of Old English *hal* "hale, whole". . .Old Norse *helge* "holy, sacred;" Old English *hælan* "to heal")[145]

The word "health" has roots in wholeness, holiness, and wellness. Be honest, how much wholeness, holiness, and wellness do you see around you in your workplace? If we are to attend to the health of patients, and not just "get our job done," then we must give of ourselves and feel with others. How can we do this when we are so busy, we see so much trauma and suffering, and the systems we work in promote disconnection and compartmentalization? Well, you will burn out if you only give and never receive. In order to provide health care and not just do our jobs, we need to continually *care for our own hearts* and *replenish our compassion.*

Stephen Trzeciak tells how he and Anthony Mazzarelli came to write a book on compassion, reviewing over 1,000 scientific abstracts and 250 research papers. Trzeciak, a self-described "research nerd," was helping his 12-year-old son with a homework problem on "what is the most pressing problem of our time?" The question gave him pause and even caused an existential crisis. Mazzarelli, the chief medical officer of Cooper University Health Care, called Trzeciak into his office and synchronistically asked him, "Does treating patients with more compassion really matter? Does caring make a difference? Does it matter in measurable ways? Put as much scientific rigor to it as you possibly can. I need you to 'science this up!'"[146] From a burnout crisis in health care workers, they became obsessed with compassion science. Their conclusion, as mentioned in the introduction, is that compassion is an evidence-based intervention.

They describe setting out "not to change people's hearts, but rather to change people's *minds*—by sharing the overwhelming scientific evidence about the effects of compassion on patient outcomes, patient safety, provider well-being, employee engagement, and organizational performance."[147] Compassion is an action, an engagement with others and the world. They make the distinction that empathy is feeling and compassion is an action, a finding that neuroscience research supports—with empathy, pain centers in the brain are activated, whereas in states of compassion, reward centers are activated. We are hardwired for compassion and compassion is a key element of what makes us human. "As compassion is defined as a response to another's pain or suffering, it is implicit that human suffering is involved," the authors maintain, and thus responding "to that suffering is the essence of what it means to be human. If one lacks compassion, one is essentially lacking humanity."[148]

This research confirms what science fiction writer Philip K. Dick postulated, that to be human means being open to another's suffering and stopping to offer help, whereas the "android" will not alter its routines and protocols. Dick's description of the android is a caution in our world of computerized treatment protocols, where we might be doing our job, but missing the suffering of the other.

> Androidization requires obedience. And most of all predictability. It is precisely when a given person's response to any given situation can be predicted with scientific accuracy that the gates are open for the wholesale production of the android lifeform.[149]

The question in contemporary health care is whether we will cultivate our compassion, which makes us human, or whether we will become machines, dehumanized androids lacking compassion. This can happen both through overzealous embrace of scientism as well as through burnout, compassion fatigue, and soul loss. We can lose touch with the heart and soul of the healer through both caring too much and caring not enough.

From Compassion Fatigue to the Compassion Revolution

> So if you stand up for caring, compassion, and the humble service of patients and communities, you are a threat to established and powerful interests.[150]
>
> ROBIN YOUNGSON

As Robin Youngson writes, there is, oddly, a lot of pressure not to care in contemporary health care. Seeing more patients, being more productive, being more "efficient," sticking rigidly to protocols, the needy computer always trying to pull you away from talking to your patient—all of these can lead to not having enough time to care. This is why I have called for a compassion revolution and a counter-curriculum as forms of "creative resistance in order to rehumanize medicine."[151]

You can read the same story of loss of idealism, demoralization, and dehumanization in the memoirs of physicians. Here is Rana Awdish describing her medical training:

> The thoughtfully designed curriculum that gifted us cadavers to dissect and learn on also disembodied us from ourselves. The lesson was: Honor these bodies before you, they are sacred and magical. And to do this you must utterly neglect your own body, your emotions, your wholeness. . . . Distance yourself from your own feelings, lest they contaminate the field.[152]

She described how, practicing in the ICU, she began to have doubts about the kind of practice we are all taught as health professionals.

> I would begin to sense a dark hole at the center of a flurry of what was otherwise highly proficient, astoundingly skillful care. I couldn't name it at first. . . . It took years of being a patient to understand that though the healing potential of knowledge is magical, it is also a lie. Medicine cannot heal in a vacuum; it requires connection.[153]

Connection is what the heart does best, whereas the mind tends to separate. Perhaps if we had more focus on compassioning with our hearts in medicine, we would not have so much burnout and compassion fatigue. Arthur Kleinman, a Harvard psychiatrist and anthropologist, also describes how he felt that the clinical curriculum was only part of what was needed to be a caring and compassionate healer.

> The clinical years of medical school fostered in me both a rising awareness of human suffering and an appreciation of the inadequacy of medical responses to the

> seemingly unlimited varieties of that suffering. . . . I became more and more efficient at eliciting the kind of information from patients that leads to an appropriate diagnosis and useful treatment. . . . But as my training progressed, I couldn't help feeling that I was losing touch with the sense of awe. . . . But that distancing also represented a kind of estrangement, an objectification that was neither necessary nor good. I had not gone into medicine so that I could turn away from the innermost feelings of care.[154]

This echoes my own feelings that I was losing something of myself, my soul, even as I was growing as a clinician. Kleinman invokes the moral nature of caring. He continues:

> Care is the glue that holds together families, communities, and societies. Care offers an alternative story of how we live and who we are. But it is being silenced in the United States and around the world, sacrificed on the altar of economy and efficiency, demanding more and more of families and health care professionals with fewer and fewer resources, and threatening to displace meaning in health care. The moral language of human experience, of people's suffering and healing—the bedrock of our common existence—is being stifled, and at worst will be lost.[155]

Kleinman notes "four seminal paradoxes" about the status of care in health care: 1) "caregiving has become increasingly peripheral to what physicians do," 2) medicine's actual caregiving is modest compared to nurses, allied health professionals, and families, yet "disregards these essential partners," 3) "there is something about medical education that actively disables students in caregiving even as it equips them with so much scientific and technical knowledge," 4) "health systems reform and the revolution in medical technology . . . have paradoxically weakened" care of the patient.[156] This is a paradox of caring, because according to Kleinman, "doctors and health care institutions still insist that caregiving is central to the practice of medicine."[157] The danger of these paradoxes is that we may think we are caring when we actually are not.

If our educational curricula can lead to loss of idealism and compassion fatigue, perhaps a different curriculum is necessary. I have used the concept of the counter-curriculum to represent what is lacking in the medical and healthcare curricula that focus solely on developing as technicians and protocol managers. The counter-curriculum is a human curriculum, a form of Continuing Human Education (CHE). John Miller has written about a "holistic curriculum" which shares many features with the counter-curriculum. The aims of the holistic curriculum are to develop: 1) wholeness/well-being, 2) wisdom and compassion, 3) awe and wonder, and 4) a sense of purpose/mastery. "Ultimately," Miller writes, "the holistic curriculum lets us realize our deeper sense of self, our soul."[158] The counter-curriculum is a holistic curriculum that aims to develop the humanity of the health professional. The counter-curriculum informs the compassion revolution, reminding us to practice being human and caring as much as being scientific and "productive."

The issue we face as physicians and health care workers is a moral one. Without our hearts of compassion, we are unable to care for ourselves or others and we become burnt out, soulless technicians. Burnout, compassion fatigue, and soul loss can seem like overwhelming problems, but take heart—your heart is filled with ever-renewing resources if you can nurture it and take the time to care. Our hearts and souls are organs of transformation that can change the suffering in our life into care, compassion, and even joy and bliss.

COMPASSIONING PRACTICE—GIVING & RECEIVING MEDITATION[159]

Imagine and visualize what the heart does on a physiological level in the body.

The heart receives (through the right atrium) the blood that has traveled throughout the entire body. This blood has the lowest oxygen content; all the tissues of the body have already absorbed oxygen from this blood—it is blue, venous blood. From the perspective of tissues, it is "bad" blood, no longer oxygen-rich. As the heart receives and accepts this "bad blood," it doesn't complain or cling to it, but gives it away, lets it go, and it passes on to the lungs. There the blood is replenished with oxygen. The heart then receives again, only this time it is the "best blood," the most oxygen-rich. Once again, however, the heart doesn't cling or hoard the goodness for itself, but gives it away to the rest of the body.

Hopefully you are seeing the metaphor of how your heart works physiologically and how you can work with suffering in your life. How much do you cling to the good? How much do you reject "bad" life experiences, which could be blessings in disguise?

Sit back for a moment, closing your eyes. Focus on what your heart is doing an average of 60 to 80 times a minute. Receiving depleted blood, giving it away; receiving replenished blood, and giving it away. Become aware of this ongoing process within you.

If you would like, focus on this same movement in your life.

Think about a situation in which you experienced suffering. Remember to step back and use some of the grounding techniques discussed in chapter 1 if you feel overwhelmed.

Allow yourself to receive it. Once you have received it, give it away again, allow it to transform, and then allow yourself to receive it again, then give it away once again. Go through this cycle of giving and receiving for as long as feels right to you. Breathe in deeply—let it flow through you; breathe out—let it go. Practice this breathing in/letting go three more times. Feel the movement of the action of your heart throughout your being. Take a deep breath, and open your eyes.

This exercise of giving and receiving shows that compassion begins within our own hearts, that we must be willing to accept both the good and the bad in order to fully feel and fully live and fully love. Transformation occurs when we accept through receiving and let go through giving.

LOVING

> Holistic health care practitioners strive to meet the patient with grace, kindness, acceptance, and spirit without condition, as love is life's most powerful healer.[160]
>
> AMERICAN HOLISTIC MEDICAL ASSOCIATION'S PRINCIPLES OF HOLISTIC MEDICINE

> One of the qualities essential of the clinician is interest in humanity, for the secret of the care of the patient is in caring for the patient.[161]
>
> FRANCIS W. PEABODY

In his 1927 article "The Care of the Patient," Peabody writes of students being taught too much about disease and not enough about caring for the patient; that medicine is both an art and a science; that the treatment of disease is impersonal and yet the care of the patient is personal; that the personal relationship is necessary for evaluation as well as treatment; and he warns about dehumanization. We are taught in medicine and health care to distance ourselves from our clients, and even if we do care about them, we are taught to have boundaries, and under no circumstances are we to *love* our patients. While it might seem radical that one of the principles of holistic medicine is love, it fits in with the idea of a compassion revolution!

For most of history, medicine was a spiritual practice. Illness and health were mysteries that the physician, the shaman, or the healer/priest of the temple of Asclepius approached with holistic techniques and interventions. They realized that they were trying to re-establish harmony and balance with nature and spirit. In turning away from the mystery of medicine, we have turned to facts and evidence. Yet with our focus on facts and evidence, we have lost sight of what is in front of us—the mystery of life, the uniqueness of the human person. We have also lost sight of love and caring in medicine.

M. Scott Peck, author of *The Road Less Traveled*, wrote that love is the "will to extend one's self for the purpose of nurturing one's own or another's spiritual growth."[162] This extending of the self of the health care professional grows out of the love that we find in the human dimension of the heart. We could even say that extending ourselves and loving others is the language of the heart. There is a spiritual element that the dimension of the heart adds to the humanity of our body, emotions, and minds. Brother Wayne Teasdale writes that part of "compassion and love is this shift from self to others . . . the realization that what matters is the interconnected whole, not just the happiness of one individual."[163]

As I reviewed in my discussion of the history of holistic medicine in my book *Re-humanizing Medicine*, the American Holistic Medical Association developed Ten Principles of Holistic Medicine. One of the principles, "The Healing Power of Love," described that "holistic health care practitioners strive to meet the patient with grace, kindness, acceptance, and spirit without condition, as love is life's most powerful healer."[164]

There are many different kinds of love and thus languages have many different words for love: *eros* (erotic), *agape* (friendship), *philia* (affection; also the root of "philosophy," which means the love of *sophia*, or wisdom), and *caritas* (charity and caring). Jean Watson, a doctor of nursing, has developed what she calls Caring Science, which focuses on *caritas* as a core value:

> As a given, caring must be grounded within a set of universal human values—kindness, concern, and Love of self and others. . . . Caritas in its original and evolved sense honors the gift of being able to give and receive with a capacity to love and appreciate all of life's diversity and its individuality within each person.[165]

For Watson, caring and *caritas* is more than an add-on to technical procedures; rather it is the essence of a profound calling and commitment to the individual and to humanity. The development and evolution of the heart moves from self to other to all. Thus, for Watson, "We move from Caritas to Communitas."[166] We can call *communitas* the creation of a loving and caring community.

Communitas & the Beloved Community

We can foster the healing power of love not just in clinical work, but in society as a whole. In caring for self & others, we must create communities of caring. An example of love informing social action and connection is what Dr. Martin Luther King Jr. called the Beloved Community:

> The core value of the quest for Dr. King's Beloved Community was agape love. Dr. King distinguished between three kinds of love: eros, "a sort of aesthetic or romantic love"; philia, "affection between friends" and agape, which he described as "understanding, redeeming goodwill for all," an "overflowing love which is purely spontaneous, unmotivated, groundless and creative" . . . "the love of God operating in the human heart." He said that "Agape does not begin by discriminating between worthy and unworthy people . . . It begins by loving others for their sakes" and "makes no distinction between a friend and enemy; it is directed toward both . . . Agape is love seeking to preserve and create community."[167]

The Beloved Community grew out of *agape* love. This, in turn, led to Dr. King's recognition of the moral value of all people, from which followed his commitment to nonviolence against others—because violence against an individual is violence against Self and the Beloved Community. Coming out of the Christian tradition, Dr. King also drew inspiration from Gandhi's work on nonviolence in India and South Africa, and he was friends with Buddhist monk Thich Nhat Hanh, who called Dr. King a Bodhisattva. As Dr. King wrote:

> In a real sense, all life is interrelated. All men are caught in an inescapable network of mutuality, tied in a single garment of destiny. Whatever affects one directly affects all indirectly. I can never be what I ought to be until you are what you ought to be, and you can never be what you ought to be until I am what I ought to be. This is the interrelated structure of reality.[168]

Communitas is a term that overlaps with the idea of the Beloved Community. Anthropologists Victor and Edith Turner and theologian Martin Buber have written about *communitas* as the breakdown of the boundaries of the individual through the arising of communal love. Catholic priest and anthropologist Gerald Arbuckle has also written about *communitas* in the development of *refounding*, which he has applied to faith communities as well as to health care institutions.[169] He describes *communitas* as either "normative" (related to structured ritual or ceremony) or "spontaneous" (occurring outside of a structured, ritual setting):

> Initiates cannot experience *communitas* if they are unwilling to struggle through chaos for the conversion of their inner selves, that is, moving from an 'I' to a 'we' ethos. Spontaneous *communitas* may or may not occur in the ritual process; it is an unplanned experience of bonding, for example the radical oneness that people feel when confronted with a natural disaster or the sight of a beautiful sunset.[170]

Can we approach burnout or soul loss in health care as opportunities for *communitas*? Instead of isolated individuals trying to do self-care on their own time, trying to put the pieces back together, could we create communities of caring, Beloved Communities that foster normative *communitas*? One solution to burnout would be to create a ritual or initiation process in health care. As Jungian analyst Robert L. Moore has written, "The burnout phenomenon among helpers is nothing . . . but . . . failed initiation."

> In contemporary culture . . . the human need for ritualization in many areas of life has not diminished. What has diminished is the availability of knowledgeable "ritual elders" who understand the archetypal human need for ritualization throughout life, and who are prepared to respond competently and effectively by providing ritual leadership to those who need it.[171]

This quote by Moore always makes me think that we need more ritual, a focus on initiation, and to build *communitas* in working with burnout, compassion fatigue, and soul loss. To do this we need love, transformation, and community. What would it look like if we had *ritual elders*, supported by institutions that value caring communities, to assist clinicians as they went through the burnout process? Remember when Chenrezig exploded into a thousand pieces and Amitābha was there to put the suffering into context and help put Chenrezig back together again? What would it look like if, instead of telling health care workers who were going through burnout and compassion fatigue to go home and do yoga and meditation, we had initiation programs where clinicians came together to form a beloved healing community?

In *Becoming Medicine: Initiation into a Living Spirituality*, we discuss *communitas* and *refounding* in the context of initiation and summarize as follows:

> *Communitas* can be thought of as a liminal state for a group in which love, devotion, and communal bonding occurs. Culture and society generally do everything they can to prevent states like *communitas* as it is a breakdown of the structure of expected social norms. *Communitas* is the energy of refounding where people feel a sense of communal oneness with each other that transcends the separation and differences that so often divide us from our brothers and sisters.[172]

So much in the practice of contemporary health care competes with community. Workers are at their desks, in their cubicles, typing away madly at their computers so that they can try to leave not too late. Where is there room or time or opportunity for *communitas*?

Loving-kindness Meditation

There is a local Tibetan Buddhist temple a few blocks from my house, and one day I heard they were holding a Chenrezig ceremony. At the ceremony, we were told that as there are infinite lifetimes, at one point every human being was our mother, and thus we should send love to all others as our mothers. This loving-kindness is called *metta* in Pali, and *bodhicitta* in Sanskrit, which means "awakened mind" and also has the connotation of care and compassion for all others. In Buddhism there is a loving-kindness practice where you cultivate the feeling of loving-kindness and then practice giving and receiving it. The 14th Dalai Lama recommends:

> Again, in order to have a sense of closeness and dearness for others, you must first train in a sense of their kindness through using as a model a person in this lifetime who was very kind to yourself and then extending this sense of gratitude toward all beings. Since, in general, in this life your mother was the closest and offered the most help, the process of meditation begins with recognizing all other sentient beings as like your mother.[173]

Not everyone had a loving mother, but most people can imagine some person who loved them unconditionally and whom they loved unconditionally. If you don't have such a person in your life, you can always imagine a religious or spiritual figure, or even a pet, or a sense of love and connection in nature.

Just as we train in medicine for various skills and protocols and memorization, so too you can train in loving-kindness. You begin with someone you feel unconditional loving-kindness toward/from, then you gradually shift out to imagining sending loving-kindness to a neutral person, then a challenging person, then to all beings. You also want to include receiving loving-kindness yourself. Some people find it easier to start with themselves, or start with another, but at some point, give yourself some loving-kindness—that is what caring for self & others is all about.

LOVING PRACTICE—LOVING-KINDNESS

Loving-kindness has a long tradition in Buddhism and the cultivation of love, caring, and compassion is found in many secular, spiritual, and religious traditions. You can call this practice loving-kindness—or if you want, *loving-careness*. I will use the term "loving-kindness" in this particular practice in honor of the tradition. You can cultivate loving-kindness as an inner resource to support you when you feel burnout, compassion fatigue, and soul loss.

If you would like to try this practice, find a comfortable posture somewhere quiet, relax your eyes, and take three deep breaths, each one deeper than the last.

Start by calling to your imagination the face of someone whom you feel a great deal of love toward. This can be anyone living or dead, a person or a pet, a child, or an adult. Focus on the feeling in your heart as you imagine this person. Imagine the feeling flowing outward toward that person as well as flowing inward to yourself.

If you lose touch with this feeling in the meditation, come back to this person to refuel yourself with loving-kindness. If you find it challenging to imagine extending loving-kindness, you can visualize a color in your heart and imagine it extending outwards to others.

Say these statements while cultivating or visualizing loving-kindness in your heart:

"May you be happy & peaceful."
"May you be safe & protected."
"May you give & receive love."

Next shift your focus toward someone you feel neutral toward. This could be a stranger you saw on the street, or a clerk at a store:

"May you be happy & peaceful."
"May you be safe & protected."
"May you give & receive love."

Now imagine someone whom you have a challenging relationship with, and send them loving-kindness:

"May you be happy & peaceful."
"May you be safe & protected."
"May you give & receive love."

Next, send loving-kindness toward yourself.

"May I be happy & peaceful."
"May I be safe & protected."
"May I give & receive love."

Lastly, send loving-kindness toward all humanity, toward all living creatures, to the entire planet:

"May we all be happy & peaceful."
"May we all be safe & protected."
"May we all give & receive love."

RELATING

> The meeting of two personalities is like the contact of two chemical substances: if there is any reaction, both are transformed . . . You can exert no influence if you are not susceptible to influence. . . . What was formerly a method of medical treatment now becomes a method of self-education, and therewith the horizon of our modern psychology is immeasurably widened. The medical diploma is no longer the crucial thing, but human quality instead.[174]
>
> CARL JUNG

> [T]he heart is far more than a pump. It plays a complex role, shaping to a significant degree our perceptions of the world through neuroendocrine roles and afferent fibers that send neural signals from heart to brain.[175]
>
> MALYNN UTZINGER

The HeartMath Institute reports that the electromagnetic field of the heart is five thousand times stronger outside the body than the electromagnetic field of the brain. They have shown that when two people sit at a conversational distance, one person's EKG (heart rhythm) can be measured within the other person's EEG (brain waves). This is an amazing finding that shows, at an electrical and electromagnetic level, that what happens in one person's heart can be measured in another person's brain, even if they are not touching each other. They call this "cardioelectromagnetic communication," and researchers have shown that in states of harmony, one person's brain can "entrain" to another person's heart, meaning that the rhythms start to mimic one another.[176]

The findings of the electrical and electromagnetic interactions between people's hearts and brain rhythms have profound implications for health care. If you are doing a technical intervention as a health care provider, but you do not have love in your heart, the other person's brain can read this and react. This also could happen in a positive way, that a clinician (or any staff member) who has love in their heart as they interact with a client can be calming and reassuring, even without saying a word.

Heart rate variability (HRV) is a measure of the balance between the sympathetic and parasympathetic tone of the body, as measured through heart rate. Healthy (or high) HRV shows more variability and micro-adjustments than does unhealthy (low) HRV. Low HRV is associated with effects on cardiovascular, neurologic, psychological, endocrine, rheumatologic, pulmonary, gastroenterological, and dermatologic systems. Interestingly, the presence of a companion dog with elderly patients has shown improvements in HRV for the person. States of anger show a lack of coherence of HRV. Relaxation shows more parasympathetic balance, represented by a greater coherence, but a state of appreciation (similar to joy or love) leads to the most coherent HRV resonance.[177] What this implies is that passive relaxation is better for the heart and health than anger is, but a state of appreciative joy and love is when the heart (and its HRV) is in the healthiest state.

We are taught that we need firm boundaries between ourselves and our clients in health care training, but the very essence of caring and nurturing others requires that we are also able to relate and connect. As Jung writes, we must be *susceptible to influence* if we want to be able to influence others. The HeartMath and HRV studies show us how we are all connected and interconnected.

Social Relationships

As discussed in chapter 2 on emotions, studies of social support after a myocardial infarction (a heart attack) have shown decreased mortality and improved health in those with good social support, or even having a pet at home.[178] The long-term Framingham study showed that those surrounded by happy people are more likely to be happy themselves, what the authors call a "dynamic spread of happiness."[179] We know that social support can benefit health, and also that a lack of social support through periods of loneliness or Adverse Childhood Experiences (ACEs) can negatively impact physical and mental health.[180]

While we often think of the heart as the organ of relating, our brains are also made for relating. Our brains have a mirror neuron network that activates when we observe others doing an action. In this sense, our brains register what we observe others doing. Neuroscientists have discussed how mirror neurons make empathy and compassion possible; that mirror neuron dysfunction might be related to autism (a lack of social relatedness); and even caution us from watching violent movies, as our brains mimic the onscreen violence.[181] We are made for relating—heart and brain!

All of My Relatives

My friend Mike Lee, ceremonial elder of the Veteran's Sweat Lodge at American Lake VA Medical Center, describes the Lakota phrase *Mitakuye Oyasin* this way:

> *Mitakuye Oyasin* means: *Mi*, "me or my," *taku*, "relative," *ye*, "I am saying this, with this breath." *Mitakuye*, "all my relatives," including: animal nation, bird nation, fish nation, creepy and crawling nation, human nation, four-legged, one legged (tree), etc. *Oyasin*, "in the oldest way

> or of ways (possible)." A greeting (male) *Aho* or *Hau Mitakuye Oyasin*. Or *Hau Mitakuye Wopila* (wopila, "this is good").[182]

We must respect cultural traditions, particularly those of groups who have suffered colonization, and always be wary of cultural appropriation. I'm not encouraging you to start using the phrase *mitakuye oyasin*, but to see if you can find and feel the concept of interrelatedness in your own heart. The meaning and worldview of this statement is worth considering as it expands the scope of our relatives beyond our blood family to the whole ecosystem of Mother Earth. Joseph Rael writes, "I pray for all my relations when we are praying in the sweat lodge. I want love. I want good rain. I want abundance for all my relations."[183] Joseph is fond of saying, "I am my brothers' and sisters' keeper," and in this he accepts all people, all animals, all plants, and Mother Earth as a relative, taking responsibility for caring for self and others.

RELATING PRACTICE—SACRED MIRROR

Psychologist John Prendergast describes a practice of "sacred mirroring" between two people, creating an "open-eyes meditative space" where attention "is nonintentional and open, alert but undirected, free of the need to accomplish or attain anything."[184] I have done this practice in my iRest teacher certification training. You can do this sitting across from another person, at a comfortable conversational distance—remember the HeartMath studies on heart/brain entrainment! You can also do this practice with yourself, looking into a mirror. You might notice waves of love and compassion, but also feelings of insecurity and self-doubt. Try to stay present with yourself and with the other person, but stay quiet, silent, and still. Here are the simple instructions that Prendergast recommends as a script and invitation:

1. Would you be interested in joining me for a period of quiet looking?

2. Let your gaze be very relaxed and soft. This is not a staring contest. Just notice your inner experience—your thoughts, feelings, and sensations—and stay with me.

3. There is no wrong way to do this and there is nothing to achieve. Welcome whatever arises. Feel free to be silent or to speak, to close your eyes at times, or to move so that you are comfortable. We can end anytime that you feel like it.[185]

This can be an intense practice. They say that the eyes are the windows to the soul and sometimes you can see into some deep places with sacred mirroring. You can also have perceptual shifts as different aspects of a person's face become more prominent, and it is not unheard of to see a person's face morph into other faces. Please debrief with your mirroring partner after the practice and share your experiences.

5

CARING FOR CREATIVITY

Wording—Drawing—Creating

Practice any art, music, singing, dancing, acting, drawing, painting, sculpting, poetry, fiction, essays, reportage, no matter how well or badly, not to get money and fame, but to experience becoming, to find out what's inside you, to make your soul grow.[186]

KURT VONNEGUT

It is in playing and only in playing that an individual child or adult is able to be creative and to use the whole personality, and it is only in being creative that the individual finds the self.[187]

DONALD WINNICOTT

CREATIVITY IS THE place where we bring ideas into form—not just pieces of art, but our actual lives. We will explore three principles of Caring for Creativity—*wording* to create stories (speaking/writing); *drawing* (and painting) to create the imagery of our lives; and *creating*.

How can we respond creatively to burnout, compassion fatigue, and soul loss? The flow of creativity is the flow of life. You can use *wording, drawing*, and *creating* to reignite the fire of the heart & soul of the healer. Creativity gets the vital life forces flowing again. When everything seems routine and mundane, remember how to play—that's how you will find your Self and your soul.

WORDING

> Words create worlds.[188]
>
> RABBI ABRAHAM JOSHUA HESCHEL

Rabbi Heschel cautions us that words can lead to creation or destruction, that our *words create worlds.* Many cultural and spiritual traditions describe the creation of the universe through sound or words. Our scientific creation story begins with a big bang. In Christianity, Genesis begins with the Spirit of God moving across the waters and the voice of God saying, "Let there be Light."[189] And, in the book of John, "In the beginning was the Word, and the Word was with God, and the Word was God."[190]

In his book *Healing the Mind Through the Power of Story*, Lewis Mehl-Madrona quotes a Lakota elder, "It's all story. There's nothing but story."[191] He then describes the four different levels of interpretation of story used by the Australian Aboriginal people: 1) the text itself; 2) relationships between people; 3) relationship of community to larger environment; 4) the spiritual reading.[192] In our lives, as well as in clinical work, we can look at people's stories through these four levels: the words themselves; the effect of those words between people; how words create (or destroy) community; and the spiritual essence embodied in the words. What Mehl-Madrona hopes is that the therapeutic use of story can help us "in transforming our vision of brain and behavior from one of defective brains (genetically or structurally) to defective stories."[193] Working with a defective story means paying attention to the words you commonly use and introducing new words into your narrative. Changing your words changes your life story and your life.

Wording can happen on the written page, but the oldest form of wording is in the sound of spoken word. Chanting and singing creates vibrations within the body and bones, much the same way that the beating heart muscle sets up electrical fields in the body. Joseph Rael writes, "The truth is this: Sound is the basis for all that is."[194] A practice that Joseph often teaches is to chant the vowel sounds: A, E, I, O, U. Joseph pronounces the vowel sounds as in Spanish: Ah, Eh, Ee, Oh, Uu (as in "you"). He will sometimes combine these with facing the five cardinal directions: Ah (east), Eh (south), Ee (west), Oh (north), Uu (center). Joseph tells us that sound creates creation.

Wording & Health

Research shows many health benefits for writing, from processing trauma to improving well-being. Studies have looked at the health benefits of expressive writing for people working with depression, anxiety, PTSD, grief, and cancer, amongst many other conditions. James Pennebaker has conducted decades of research on the benefits of writing, which he summarizes in his book with Joshua Smyth, *Opening Up by Writing It Down: How Expressive Writing Improves Health and Eases Emotional Pain*. I also like Louise DeSalvo's book *Writing as a Way of Healing*, which opens with her words, "Writing has helped me heal. Writing has changed my life. Writing has saved my life."[195]

Writing can also be used for working with burnout in health care professionals and trainees. For instance, Kulchar and Haddad published a set of practices for working with burnout during the COVID-19 pandemic that includes writing activities among them.[196] A small study by Narayan, Stern, and Fornari found that fourth-year medical students who participated in an elective health humanities course that utilized reflective writing had lower rates of burnout after the course.[197]

During my fourth year of medical school, I took an elective in narrative medicine and medical humanities at University of Illinois Chicago (UIC). We read papers on medical humanities, wrote reflective poems about our medical education experience, and an essay on a medical writer. The words just flowed out of me as I reflected back on different experiences in my education. The strange thing about medicine is that we are thrown into the most existentially extreme life-and-death situations with patients, and yet there was no time or space or encouragement to reflect and process the emotional aspects of becoming a physician.

One of my first poems, "I stare out,"[198] was published in the UIC medical humanities journal, *Body Electric*. It must have resonated with others, as it was re-published five times, including in an academic article and a book on medical student poetry. I have continued journaling and writing poetry throughout my life and I find it a necessary part of my medical practice. I include narrative and memoir elements in my professional writing. I draw inspiration from the work of Rebecca Solnit, who blends memoir, scholarly research, beautiful poetic prose, and activism and engagement with the world. I have continued to support the medical and health humanities through my work with Jonathan McFarland and the wonderful international team at The Doctor as a Humanist. We encourage writing and the arts as ways of reflecting on medical practice and health care education.

Through my interest in writing, medical humanities, and physician health, I attended a number of the Australasian Doctors' Health conferences in New Zealand and Australia. It was there that I met Hilton Koppe, and we put on a workshop in 2017 in Melbourne, Australia, on The Healer's Journey, building on Joseph Campbell's hero's journey concept. Hilton has just published a wonderful work of narrative medicine filled with sorrow, humor, and wisdom, *One Curious Doctor: A Memoir of Medicine, Migration and Mortality*. As Hilton succinctly writes, "I start writing about being a doctor. As my pen gives voice to the unspeakable—despair, grief, fear, betrayal—stories and poems emerge. The writing process is surprisingly helpful."[199] Medical memoir is a persistent genre because medicine places us at the edge of health and illness, the edge of life and death, and into madness and trauma; doctors and other health care professionals have long felt the need to document their journeys to the end of night in search of a new dawn after experiencing dark nights of the soul.

WORDING PRACTICE—WRITING YOUR LIFE

I encourage you to consider making wording a part of your ongoing Continuing Human Education. Here are a few different practices:

Journaling about your day: This could be done in stream-of-consciousness style, writing about whatever arises. You can also focus on specific things, like choosing the most stressful and the best part of the day and writing out those events. Much of the research on the health benefits of writing focuses on emotional processing, so see if you can elaborate your feelings, thoughts, and bodily sensations as well as the objective events. Writing helps you integrate the inner and outer worlds.

Writing the narrative of stressful events:[200] This is different than journaling because you are telling a story. I did this in medical school and residency—after a stressful situation that was hard to shake, I found it helpful to write it down like a story, remembering as many details as possible. Just as when working with a dream, you may find elements you forgot, and things might make more sense to you after you write it out.

If you'd like some great examples of this technique, here are some of my favorites: My mate Hilton Koppe, has written his narrative in the book *One Curious Doctor* (mentioned on the opposite page), and his website lists other material on writing for doctors.[201] My good friend Chris Smith, has written *Be a Good Story*, which blends writing prompts for your story within a thread of his life stories of learning.[202] I also like the Transformative Language Arts Network as a general resource for writing for personal and collective transformation.

Write a poem: Poetry is a great way to process stress and emotions because you can bypass the logical mind and just flow with the images, emotions, and connections. I always say that anyone can write poetry because it is simply writing without worrying about punctuation. You can also play around with rhymes, rhythms, and patterns as a way of creating a structure for your emotions.

I share examples of poetry on my website.[203] Examples from my medical and psychiatric education are: "I stare out," "it is internship year," "I Remember," and "And What Can Really Be Controlled in Life?"

Connecting past and present: Think about something you loved to do as a child, or what you wanted to do when you grew up. Write from memory of your perspective as a child. Pay special attention to your feelings of joy, vitality, and excitement. Now consider how much joy, vitality, and excitement you have in your present life. How can you connect those feelings of youthful enthusiasm from the past and bring them into your life now?

Gratitude Practice: Try writing about three things every day that you are grateful for in your life. A gratitude practice can really shift your perspective from the negative to the positive. For instance, when my melanoma surgery was delayed for hours and I was waiting in pre-op, instead of getting upset at the personal inconvenience to me, I kept reminding myself to be grateful for the fact that I was not in need of urgent surgery and thus was a lower priority for an operating room.

Chanting: This is an ancient technique that is beginning to be researched for health benefits. For instance, see the work of Jill Bormann with her Mantram Repetition Program.[204] Robert Gass and Kathleen Brehony's book ***Chanting: Discovering Spirit in Sound*** also reviews research and practices. All you really need to practice chanting is to choose a word or phrase and repeat it at your own pace, feeling the sound and vibrations throughout your whole body. You can add music or listen to recordings of singing and chanting, such as by Robert Gass and On Wings of Song, or Bill Laswell's Sacred System albums and his other collaborations. A couple of my favorite chanting albums are Ravi Shankar and George Harrison's ***Chants of India*** and ***Rain of Blessings: Vajra Chants*** by Lama Gyurme and Jean-Philippe Rykiel.

DRAWING & PAINTING

We can draw what is out in the world or we can draw from inner images. Drawing brings together the inner and outer: when we look without, we are drawing on the outer world, and when we look within, we are drawing on the inner world. Balancing inner and outer is a healing power of drawing.

In *Drawing on the Right Side of the Brain*, Betty Edwards explores the perspectives of the left brain (analytical) and right brain (creative). She argues that we need both sides working in tandem in order to be fully balanced human beings:

> The ideal role of the right hemisphere . . . is to provide access to the deepest levels of one's true experience . . . The ideal role for the left hemisphere is to be an articulate spokesperson for all the information that comes up from the right and to discriminate between what's important and what is merely trivial. Each mode of thinking is incomplete without the other. You need access to both hemispheres to be whole.[205]

This understanding of right brain/left brain is important in health care as it can be a metaphor for the art and science of medicine. (We have already considered the work of Iain McGilchrist earlier in the book on this topic and will do so again in the next chapter.) We want to have both of these modes of thinking and being in order to be whole ourselves and to meet the whole person we work with. Thus, one of the ways we can care for creativity is to draw and paint and sculpt, to work with forms and images in order to express that which is within us and to harmonize inside and outside.

Painting

Painting is another way to care for your creativity. Jung used the term "active imagination" for engaging with characters and images from dreams and imaginings as a way of bringing forth deeper knowledge of ourselves from our unconsciousness into our consciousness. Jung developed this method during a time of great stress and deep soul searching after his break with Freud.

Jung's written inner dialogues from his 1913–1932 journals were posthumously published in *The Black Books*. In the illuminated manuscript he called *Liber Novus*, or *The Red Book*, Jung elaborated upon his written inner dialogues by adding illustrations and mandalas. *The Black Books* and *The Red Book* were published years after Jung's death, although he often referenced the contents and shared parts of them with colleagues and patients. Through writing, drawing, and painting, Jung worked through his dark night of the soul and uncovered the inspirations that kept him busy for the rest of his life. He also began to build small stone structures, as he had when he was a child, and eventually he built his own personal retreat center, Bollingen Tower. Jung didn't consider himself an artist or that he was "making art"—he was doing inner therapeutic work. Similarly, you don't have to try to create art, but simply express yourself.

Art Therapy

> Art heals by accepting the pain and doing something with it.[206]
>
> SHAUN MCNIFF

Jungian psychology influenced the emergence of the field of art therapy. Jung used a wide range of creative practices, as Shaun McNiff points out.

> Jung made use of a wide array of expressive activities: dream work, drawing mandalas every morning, writing, gathering stones, symbolic play, yoga exercises, dramatic personification, dialogues with the figure of Philemon and other images, active fantasy, painting pictures of visions, hewing stone, building imaginary castles and villages, contemplating nature, and enacting personal rituals.[207]

Art therapy became a formal profession in the mid-20th century. Farrelly-Hansen describes art therapy as having "a high tolerance of chaos, for both destructive and constructive aspects of the creative act," and that the "urge to create is understood as a bodily instinct."[208] Art and art therapy bring together pain and joy, suffering and bliss, and creation and destruction. As a *bodily instinct*, creating stirs the soul and makes us human. As McNiff writes, "Art and creativity are the soul's medicines—what the soul uses to minister to itself, cure its maladies, and restore its vitality."[209] Art is an antidote for burnout, compassion fatigue, and soul loss! We can use the *costs of caring* as raw materials for art therapy, as McNiff tells us:

> The most difficult situations have always presented the greatest opportunities for transformation, both collective and individual. Without conflict and pain, one never reaches the depths of being, the most intense and formative places. So rather than blunting the awareness of my conflicts through avoidance, I try to stay close to them, to directly engage their power to transform . . . Artists throughout history have shown that creativity comes from conflict . . . It is the artist, the creator, who can teach us how to engage with the energy of conflict.[210]

I have used art (by which I mean creative work and play) throughout my life. I have found that the most rewarding creating comes from when I am either overflowing with inspiration or when I am in the depths of a dark night of the soul. Often an image will present itself in my imagination, or something from a dream will stick in my mind. During dark times, I just enter deeper into the darkness. Maybe I will paint a thick layer of black or white paint on a canvas or piece of paper. Then I will put drops of different colors on top, and then I have a spray bottle that I spray on the paint. I watch the movement of colors. Sometimes I will take a snapshot with my phone of different transitional stages. I stare into the paint and see what wants to arise from it. This method does not control the results, but rather involves giving oneself up to the internal depths and the play of color. I have a selection of my paintings featured on my website, davidkopacz.com.

Art can be our burnout medicine, our compassion fatigue medicine, our *soul's medicine*. Hippocrates said, "Life is short, and Art long; the crisis fleeting; experience perilous, and decision difficult. The physician must not only be prepared to do what is right himself, but also to make the patient, the attendants, and externals cooperate."[211] We can turn to art—as a practice of soul medicine, a practice of healing, and a practice of living. This kind of art is not about producing an aesthetic product, but rather is the practice of being fully human.

DRAWING & PAINTING PRACTICES— BECOMING AN ARTIST OF YOUR LIFE

These practices are not necessarily about becoming an artist, other than maybe becoming an artist of your life. The three things you need for this practice are: space, time, and materials. Space includes both physical and interpersonal space. To connect to your inner domain, you need a space that is free of distraction and observation for a period of time. It doesn't have to be long, even just 15–30 minutes. Time is often the most challenging. Julia Cameron, in her book *The Artist's Way*, encourages people to set an "artist date,"[212] setting aside time and a plan of a trip to a museum or somewhere for inspiration, or it could be setting a time for you to do drawing and painting practices.

Materials can be as simple as a pen or pencil and some printer paper, or purchasing colored pens or pencils, or some inexpensive paints such as watercolors or acrylics, and art paper. Watercolors tend to bleed and blend. Acrylics can be more expensive (although you can find deals on sets) but allow more precision. I like to use acrylics and then use a spray bottle to make them flow more like watercolors for the background, and then use undiluted acrylics for more precise lines after the background dries. There are many different techniques you can use to create different effects. I have even bought gallons of mis-tinted paint from a hardware store for a couple of dollars, then made my own frames with craft wood and plywood and primed it before painting. One technique I played around with for a while was adding layers of latex paint one on top of the other on a primed plywood "canvas" with a handmade frame that created a kind of shallow bowl. Then I would bounce a tennis ball on the thick paint, and it would make splash craters of color that reminded me of the craters of the moon. The point is, be creative and let your materials guide you as much as you work with them toward whatever vision you have in mind. Sometimes I start with a vision of what I'd like to create, but often I just listen to the materials and see what arises. As I am not a very skilled artist, I always work to compromise between a vision and what emerges.

Consider these suggestions, and if they do not click for you, feel free to come up with other practices.

Non-dominant hand drawing: Use your non-dominant hand to sketch. You can try to draw "things," or you can just let your hand move and enjoy the feelings of movement and creation.

Drawing upside down: This is a technique Betty Edwards writes about. Take a picture of whatever you want to draw and turn it upside down—this way you are able to just draw what is there instead of over-thinking it.

Scribble drawing: Let your hand make loops and scribbles. Next look at it as you would look at a cloud or woodgrain pattern—look for faces, shapes, objects. Next, add color through drawing or painting.

Drawing or sketching what you see: This is what most people think of when they think of drawing, but it takes a little skill or some adventurous creativity to develop your own style if you do not have technical skills.

Painting: This can be as technically precise or spontaneously playful as you like. I am not above using my fingers as I like to have an intimate relationship with the feel of the paint and the colors. As you play around with painting, you can get different-size brushes for different effects.

CREATING

Life is creation. The soul comes to life through creating. Yet so much of life is taken up by duties and responsibilities that we never get to what really matters. That is one way of looking at burnout—we get so busy doing things in the world that we forget to tend our inner flame; we get so immersed in helping others that we neglect our inner world and creativity. When we don't tend to our souls, they wander away from us while we are sweating on the assembly line of life. As Rumi wrote, "The soul is here for its own joy."[213] What is the joy that your soul is here for? What is that thing that you must do in your life?

Joseph Rael (Beautiful Painted Arrow) writes, "We do not exist."[214] He elaborates on this strange statement: "When I say that we do not exist, I mean that the only time we truly exist is when we are reaching and being our highest potential . . . At any other time, we are not contributing either to ourselves or to humanity."[215] This statement, that we do not exist, except when we are *reaching or being our highest potential*, captures the essence of creating. The effort to keep things the same actually takes us away from ourselves. The oldest, ancient story is that the soul longs to be born anew in the present moment. Beautiful Painted Arrow says that we are already born healers.

> We are already born shamans, we just forget it as we grow older. Being a shaman is being a healer, but it isn't you who heals, it is *Wah-Mah-Chi*, Breath, Matter, Movement. The job of a shaman is to be a "hollow bone." You are just a hollow bone that Breath, Matter, Movement flows through.[216]

We are healers by creating space within us for healing energy to flow through. What we are creating is not the filling of ourselves, or being full of ourselves, but creating the space for that which spontaneously fills us when we are empty and not existing—and then we are truly in the present moment and we remember that we are already healers.

Living Our Inner Genius

Storyteller Michael Meade has written about the soul and the ancient Roman idea of "genius," our guiding inner nature, a concept I mentioned briefly back in chapter 1. Meade sees that, as moderns, we realize that "something meaningful has gone missing and must be sought for again." "The inner genius," he continues, "is our inherent and indelible connection to the otherworld of great imagination, original thought and endless renewal. . . . [it is] both ancient and immediate at the same time."[217]

> When the daily world becomes a state of chaos and constant turmoil, it is time to turn back to the mythic imagination that resides deep within the soul. For there is a myth at the heart of things and a core of imagination residing in the heart of each person. Part of the secret of life is that each soul carries a primary imagination and reservoir of essential ideas that can help us make sense of the fleeting world. Imagination is the deepest power of the human soul and mythic imagination helps make meaning of all that happens in the world, even as it helps reveal inner meanings and genuine purpose in the heart of each person.[218]

Meade's descriptions of chaos and constant turmoil sound a lot like burnout, the emptiness of compassion fatigue, and soul loss. The human reality of suffering—for us as healers as well as for our patients—can be a source of pain and despair, but it can also be a call to adventure, an initiation into deeper levels of wisdom as healers. The *costs of caring* remind us to reconnect to our roots, to our origin story of why we were called to become healers in the first place. Suffering reminds us that we must go back to the source of endless renewal within ourselves, that we must enter into dialogue with our soul, and that we must reacquaint ourselves with our inner genius. Suffering can challenge us to let go of our depleted myth of being all-powerful, all-caring, all-knowing, sending us back to searching for the ground of ourselves, the ground of our being. It is there that we pick up the thread to re-weave the story of our Self because of the story our soul and inner genius is whispering to us of what we can be.

What if we are only truly ourselves when we are creating? In all creating, we are creating our Selves. We create our lives every moment. The material we use is our bodies, emotions, thoughts. Inspiration comes from our hearts, creativity, intuition, and spirit. Life is a creative endeavor and we are all artists and poets of our lives.

Poiesis: Knowing by Creating

In their book *Nature-Based Expressive Arts Therapy*, Sally Atkins and Melia Snyder describe how "a nature-based orientation to expressive arts returns us to our imagination, our intuition, our physical bodies and the body of the Earth."[219] In this sense, art is integrative, bringing together the inner world of self and the outer world of nature. They write of the Greek word *poiesis*, meaning "to know by creating," which leads to a reciprocal relationship in which "we are both shaping and shaped by the world in which we live."[220] Creating arises from embodiment or the coming together of body, mind, soul, and Earth. Creating is both an expression of soul and a pathway for reconnecting with soul.

Related to *poesis* is *mythopoesis*—the creation of myth. Myth in this sense is not what is false, but rather that truth that we can only tell by leaving the logical world and entering into the mythical. James Hillman developed a psychology that drew on images—imaginal psychology. He wrote of the *mythopoetic imagination*, which speaks through images, mythology, and poetry about our deepest truths. In *Healing Fiction*, Hillman writes about the role that imagination and narrative play in health and illness. More specifically, he looked at the imaginative narratives that underlay the theories of Freud, Jung, and Adler. Rather than looking for childhood traumas or reductionistic biological explanations for mental health and illness, Hillman describes "a psychology that assumes a poetic basis of mind."

> By placing depth psychology within a poetical and rhetorical cosmos . . . I essayed a psychology of the soul that is also a psychology of the imagination, one which takes its point of departure neither in brain physiology, structural linguistics, nor analyses of behavior, but in the process of imagination.[221]

Jung described a sense of soul loss and mythic disorientation that led him to develop the process of "active imagination." This occurred around 1913 after he published his book on the hero myth, which led to his break from his mentor, Freud, over Jung's view that there was wisdom in the unconscious and that even the suffering of neurosis carried within it a seed of transformation. Jung thought to himself:

> "Now you possess a key to mythology and are free to unlock all the gates of the unconscious psyche." But then . . . the question arose of what, after all, I had accomplished. I had explained the myths of peoples of the past; I had written a book about the hero, the myth in which man has always lived. But in what myth does man live nowadays? "But then what is your myth—the myth in which you do live?" At this point the dialogue with myself became uncomfortable, and I stopped thinking. I had reached a dead end.[222]

This dead end eventually led to a flood of spontaneous images that Jung spent years working with in *The Red Book*. Sometimes we have to lose the plot of the lives we think we should be living. It is disorienting and frightening to not know what underlying myth, narrative, or poesis is unfolding in our lives. The writers we have been visiting with comfort us with the knowledge that there is an inner guiding force in our lives, and when we connect with this inner guiding force, we are aligned with our calling as well as connected with the Earth. Imagination, poetry, and poesis are all ways that we can find the thread of our authentic narrative, the story your soul is trying to tell through your life.

CREATING PRACTICE—CREATING YOUR STORY

Some of the oldest stories are creation stories—stories about where we humans started—about how we often lose track of our *original instructions* and go astray, and about remembering where we are trying to go. There is a story in Rumi's *Masnavi* about a man from Baghdad who dreams of a treasure buried in Egypt. He travels there and begins to dig, but is apprehended by the police. When he tells a policeman that he was in Cairo digging in the ground because of a dream, the policeman laughs at him for traveling all that way for a dream. The policeman says he had a similar dream of buried treasure in Baghdad, but he was never fool enough to chase after a dream. As the policeman describes the house in Baghdad, where the treasure is buried, the man recognizes it is his own house where he first had the dream about treasure in Cairo. He returns to Baghdad and unearths the dreamed of treasure buried in his own home, exclaiming, "The water of life is here. I'm drinking it. But I had to come this long way to know it!"[223]

We often lose touch with our treasure and we may have to travel far to remember that it was hidden right under our feet, that we contain it within ourselves. We can use the wreckage of our lives—our burned-out shells, our empty and bruised hearts, that empty place where our souls used to be—we can use these materials to *re-member* ourselves, just as Chenrezig was re-membered to have a thousand arms to better touch suffering.

If you feel overwhelmed with this practice, go back to grounding—or better yet, work with some paint or drawing and work your emotions onto paper. Then return to this creating your story practice. You can always seek a therapist's support if it becomes too overwhelming.

Begin where you are.

Find your burnout. Where is it located? What does it feel like? Don't just think about it—feel it.

Drop into the emptiness of your compassion fatigue, into the emptiness of your heart.

Drop into that hole where your soul used to be.

This is an ancient journey. Dante started off in a dark wood, then he dropped down to hell, worked his way up to purgatory, and then finally made it to heaven.

Allow yourself to enter into the wreckage of your life.

For a moment, just witness it, like Chenrezig in the moment of exploding into a thousand pieces before being put back together. These pieces are the raw material of your life. They are the ashes from which the phoenix of your renewed story will arise.

Sit in the stillness and silence of the wreckage of your life and sink deeper into it.

See if anything stirs.

See if any last little bit of life is there: a seed, a smoldering, a small light, a few pages of the book of your life, some renewal in this wasteland of your life.

With these raw materials, try writing or drawing or painting.

Start with the wreckage of the wasteland and then see what might emerge.

Allow the images to work on you; you don't need to work on them, you don't need to make them do anything.

Allow the images to arise because the soul and inner genius is the source of these images, these landscapes of the soul that you are traveling.

After you have sat in this place of the destruction of the old, start to work on the creation of the new, incorporating whatever you find at hand.

Begin again, as you have a thousand times before; begin again to feel, to hope, to imagine.

Allow your own inner healer to start to heal you—to clean the wound, to bring the edges together, to activate your soul.

Write, draw, paint, create. See what arises, something always will. Write, draw, paint, create. Breathe. Breathe. Breathe.

6

CARING FOR INTUITION

Dreaming—Visioning—Receiving

> **intuit** (v.) "to tutor," from Latin *intuit-*, past participle stem of *intueri* "look at, consider". . . Meaning "to perceive directly without reasoning, know by immediate perception . . . "[224]

IN BURNOUT AND compassion fatigue, we can lose our vision, we can lose our dreams, we can feel cut off from receiving the vitality and wisdom of our souls. When we reach the limits of what our conscious minds can make sense of, it is time to open up your intuition to receive dreams and visions that can give you a new orientation in life. Intuition is a direct *sense of knowing* that is not intellectual or linear. We will explore three fundamental attributes of Caring for Intuition—*dreaming* (interpreting the symbols of dreams, myths, and signs), *visioning* (seeing connections below the surface of things), and *receiving* (becoming a conduit for intuitive knowledge).

Intuition is a natural human ability, but we lose touch with it through our excessive focus on objectivity and linear thought. McGilchrist has two chapters reviewing the research on intuition in his book

The Matter With Things, finding that intuition is a function of the right hemisphere.

> Intuition appears to be something that, while inevitably fallible, is often more reliable, much quicker, and capable of taking into account many more factors, than explicit reasoning, including factors of which we may not even be consciously aware . . . The attempt to replace it with rules and procedures is a typical left hemisphere response to something it does not understand—a response that is, alas, powerfully destructive. We inhabit a world in which reason is needed more than ever before, yet in which reason is so narrowly conceived that it drives out true understanding. For that we would have had to learn respect for the power of intuition, not as opposed to reason, but as both grounding it, and the means for it to fulfill its potential in making judgments in life.[225]

If you are too much in your mind, your ego, or the left hemisphere, you won't notice intuition. Remember the study by Chabris and Simons on the gorilla on the basketball court or in the radiology image from chapter 3? When we are very focused on a linear, intellectual task such as counting or scanning for certain things, this can block out other things that we were not expecting to see. Intuition can complement intellect and logic by going outside the box.

Here is a clinical example. If we are just ticking off boxes and going through checklists, we can miss nuances. As a psychiatrist, when I ask someone if they are having suicidal thoughts, I am listening to more than whether they say "yes" or "no." I am listening to how it is said and how fast it is said. I am also listening to what is not said. This kind of listening is what Reik called "listening with the third ear" in his book *Listening with the Third Ear: The Inner Experience of a Psychoanalyst*. The third ear is using intuition to listen to everything around the words. Reik would say that listening with the third ear is using intuition for the therapist to access their unconscious to better understand the client. Assessing for suicide risk is as much asking the right questions as it is learning how to hear both the answers that are spoken as well as what is unspoken.

Learning psychotherapy, particularly psychotherapies that work with the unconscious, is really about honing our intuition. When I teach psychotherapy to trainees, I focus on psychotherapy as primarily a practice of listening and connecting. Technical interventions should grow out of deeply being with clients rather than from a manual, a protocol, or a theory. This is one of the most challenging things to teach doctors, that psychotherapy is about listening and being with people. Our culture in general focuses on actions and quick fixes, and young psychiatrists in particular are primed for quick action after working in the emergency department, rather than focusing on slow understanding.

Intuition can be cultivated by slowing down, paying attention, and listening. The prophet Elijah did not find God in the wind or the earthquake or the fire, but in a "still small voice."[226]

DREAMING

Dreams are illustrations from the book your soul is writing—your life. Cultures around the world have valued dreams for intuitive understanding. Dreams are found throughout the Holy Books—the Bible, the Torah, the Qur'an, and other religious texts. Psychology, too, particularly in the early 20th century with Freud and Jung, turned to dreams to reveal the unconscious and deeper levels of Self.

Dreams speak in the language of symbols—metaphors of image and meaning. From a literal perspective, symbols seem illogical and meaningless, but there is a deeper meaning in them. Dreams have a kind of felt sense—a different language of meaning. Dream language is not often taught in contemporary Western society.

A famous example of a scientific breakthrough in a dream was the discovery of the benzene chemical ring structure. Kekulé had been working on a scientific problem when he dozed off and saw molecules dancing before his eyes, which transformed into snakes and one of the snakes bit its own tail. The circular ring structure solved the problem of how the known components of benzene could fit together. Kekulé later recounted, "As if by a flash of lightning

I awoke; and this time also I spent the rest of the night in working out the consequences of the hypothesis. Let us learn to dream . . . then perhaps we shall find the truth."[227]

One of Jung's techniques for interpreting dreams was to see every character in the dream as an unconscious aspect of yourself. To this end, he recommended going toward rather than away from what scares you in your dreams or what you fear, which represents your "shadow," the unacknowledged aspects of yourself that come out in a dark way. Here is an example of a dream I had years ago that took a transformative turn when I applied this principle.

The Dream of the Black Dog[228]

I am walking across a plain. A solid, small, but fierce-looking black dog-like creature comes bounding toward me across the plain. The dog has a shimmering quality, but also seems to be absorbing light so that it is difficult to focus on clearly. My temptation is to turn and run, but there is nowhere to go and the dog is much faster. I stand my ground. The "dog" comes toward me and starts a kind of growl, barking and jumping around me. It feels threatening to me, but I take a deep dream breath and say to it, "What do you want of me?"

Instantly, the dog calms down, starts wagging its tail and runs a few steps, looks back, runs a few steps, and looks back. It wants me to follow. The dog is very heavy and dense, absorbing light, like something from another planet or another dimension. I run to try to keep up as it goes up over the crest of a hill. I can see down into an ocean cove where a pod of beautiful, golden-colored, whale-like creatures are stranded on the beach. The dog and I run down to the beach. Between the two of us, we are able to push and roll the golden whale creatures back into the sea. They are very grateful and begin cavorting about in the waves offshore, seemingly thanking us and waving goodbye.

I often draw upon the images of the golden creatures and their gratitude. I remind myself when faced with an initially fearful situation, to try to shift from fear to curiosity. Just think about what I would have missed if I ran from the black dog or refused to follow it. It can be challenging to face what we fear, but we never know what gifts are awaiting us in the unknown.

DREAMING PRACTICE—WORKING WITH YOUR DREAMS

Robert Johnson gives an outline for working with dreams in his book *Inner Work: Using Dreams and Active Imagination for Personal Growth.* He recommends breaking down dream interpretation into four steps:

1. Making associations
2. Connecting dream images to inner dynamics
3. Interpreting
4. Doing rituals to make the dream concrete[229]

You can enhance your memories of dreams by writing down as much as you remember when you first wake up. Even if you wake up in the middle of the night, you can jot down in a journal or on a piece of paper, for instance: orphanage, having lunch together, building a bridge, wanting to support the kids.

Later you can fill in the details around these key images or themes. With this first elaboration, certain images, symbols, or events may seem more relevant to you, more interesting, or more disturbing. You can then work with those as you make associations.

Johnson's first step is mapping out your immediate associations to each image element. Associations are your first, automatic, intuitive, or reflexive thoughts and feelings as you look at the dream. You want to do this before your mind starts trying to analyze and reduce the dream to a specific meaning. For instance, with an image of a blue door on a red house, you could map out your associations to "blue," "door," "red," and "house." He encourages coming up with a few associations for each image. For instance, for "blue," he gives examples someone might come up with: "cool, detached," "sad," "my favorite sweater," "blew, blown away," "true blue," and "clarity."[230]

Johnson's second step is to "take the dream inward" and to connect the associations to the images with your inner emotions and processes. You can take the perspectives of different characters in the dream and see how they all might represent inner parts of yourself that are trying to work something out. It is at this level that you might start looking at more complex meanings to the whole dream, not just your associations to different parts of it.

In Johnson's third step, you put all the pieces together from the associations and how they relate to deeper patterns and meanings in your life and look at what the dream might be representing or be trying to tell you. Jungians look at dreams as guides trying to help you learn and grow.

In Johnson's fourth step, he recommends engaging in rituals or creative processes to act out or represent the dream in physical reality. This could be through acting out movements, painting or drawing, sculpting, or doing what was happening in the dream (within reason of course). For instance, if you have a dream about gardening, go out and get your hands in the dirt. If you have a dream about walking in the woods, take a walk in the woods. Bring a journal if you do this and try writing about your experience. Johnson views this last step as an important part of making the unconscious conscious.

VISIONING

> All visions are always present. A vision is what a visionary is seeing. . . . When we see visions, they enter perceptual reality. In perceptual reality, the visionary is seeing something in front of him or her that is now available to be perceived by a perceiver, who has allowed himself now to perceive.
>
> A vision is the soul drinking light. It starts with descending light, falling like rain. . . . The visionary transformation happens in the act of perception . . . It has the quality of "heaven is here now." What you want to achieve is here now, ready, given.[231]
>
> JOSEPH RAEL (BEAUTIFUL PAINTED ARROW)

Visioning is learning to use our intuition in our lives.[232] You've heard the saying, "A picture is worth a thousand words." This is the truth of visioning and intuition—an image contains information that can be understood quicker than it can be explained. A vision is seeing through your intuition, which is different than seeing through your physical eyes. When we are visioning, we are "seeing" in a different way; we are sensitive to patterns, to the connections between things, not only the things themselves.

In the religious texts of the world, people hear the voice of God, meet angels and spirits, and have all sorts of visionary experiences. Indigenous traditions, historically and in the present day, practice seeking visions as a process of spiritual growth, as an initiation rite, or to gather intuitive guidance in relation to big questions or problems.

In *Becoming Medicine*, we have a chapter on "Becoming a Visionary." We examine Joseph's teachings as well as modern visionaries like Carl Jung and Henry Corbin. Joseph makes a distinction between two realities, *ordinary reality* and *non-ordinary reality*. Non-ordinary reality is the place of visions; Joseph was able to spontaneously go into this realm as a child, and then he received further training from the Elders at Picuris Pueblo as he was growing up. Much of his work reminds us that we are all born visionaries; we just have to slow down and open ourselves to receiving visions. Visioning is like a waking dream—it is a flash of insight that helps us understand ourselves and our place in the universe.

Henry Corbin was born in France in 1903 and studied esoteric Islam and Sufism. He traveled to Iran in 1939 and the outbreak of World War II stranded him there for six years. Perhaps his being stuck between, in a liminal place, contributed to his interest in the *'ālam al-mithāl*, the "place of visions." What Corbin learned in his studies was that visions occur in a place between the spiritual world and the material world, the "world of archetypal Images through and in which *Spirits are corporealized and bodies are spiritualized*."[233] He distinguished between the make-believe of fantasy that occurs in our minds and the journey to the place of visions, or the Earth of visions, the *'ālam al-mithāl*.

> Here we shall not be dealing with imagination in the usual sense of the word: neither with fantasy, profane

> or otherwise, nor with the organ which produces imaginings identified with the unreal; nor shall we even be dealing exactly with what we look upon as the organ of esthetic creation. We shall be speaking of an absolutely basic function, correlated with a universe peculiar to it, a universe endowed with a perfectly "objective" existence and perceived precisely through the Imagination."[234]

In a similar way to Jung, who instructed his clients on using *active imagination* for therapeutic purposes, Corbin also wrote about *active imagination*,[235] but as an organ of perception and a vehicle to travel to the place of visions where matter is spiritualized and spirit is materialized. "The organ of this universe," Corbin wrote, "is the active Imagination; it is the *place* of theophanic visions, the scene on which visionary events and symbolic histories *appear* in their true reality."[236]

Joseph Rael also speaks of a place of visions: non-ordinary reality. The shamanic journey to non-ordinary reality shares features with the Sufis' journey that Corbin describes. Both Corbin and Joseph describe the universe as a place of continual creation that emanates from the *'ālam al-mithāl*, or non-ordinary reality, respectively. Visionary reality is necessary to bring reality into being and it is also where we can find a sense of *living spirituality*—you could say it is the place where we find our souls when we lose them. Without our soul's connection to the place of visions, we feel deadened, dispirited, even dehumanized. Joseph tells us that visioning helps us as our "fullest potential comes when we get a flash of light. We reach a peak experience at which point we've broken through to a new level of being . . . a new level of awareness. We have touched the source of our inspiration."[237]

How is it that we make this journey? How can we connect with our soul's fullest potential? Joseph tells us that we can reach living spirituality through ceremony, or ritual practices, what he calls "crying for a vision."

> Ceremony is the way to do this. It gives us these powers. Ceremony works because it is crying for a vision. By

> crying for a vision, I mean that the soul is longing for light, so it can drink it in and thus fulfill its nature. If light—vision—is lacking, there is sadness.[238]

Once you get a vision, you need to bring it into reality somehow. This is what Joseph Rael did when he had a vision of a Sound Peace Chamber—a circular structure, half above ground, half below ground, with men and women sitting in a circle, chanting for world peace. Over 60 Chambers have been constructed around the world, and he received a letter of recognition from the United Nations for his work on world peace.

Jung's *Red Book* is an exercise in active imagination, an example of how he continually brought his visions into the written word and in colorful images.[239] Jung's journey begins by him calling to his lost soul. "My soul, my soul, where are you? Do you hear me? I speak, I call you—are you there? I have returned, I am here again. . . . After long years of long wandering, I have come to you anew."[240] Jung learned that the language of the soul was different than his previous academic learning, as "the soul is everywhere that scholarly knowledge is not."[241] Jung's exploration of inner images through active imagination laid the groundwork for the grand work of the rest of his life.

> The years when I was pursuing my inner images were the most important in my life—in them everything essential was decided. It all began then; the later details are only supplements and clarifications of the material that burst forth from the unconscious, and at first swamped me. It was the *prima materia* for a lifetime's work.[242]

For Jung, first came the overwhelming flood of images and emotions. Secondarily, he developed the process of working to capture the images and visions in words, drawings, and paintings. For most people, images and visioning do not come automatically, but need to be cultivated through the practice Jung called active imagination—allowing the images to speak for themselves.

VISIONING PRACTICE—JOURNEYING TO THE PLACE OF VISIONS

Institutions have vision statements these days, but these visions are often not embodied in reality. Can we discover our own vision statements—ones that have meaning to us in our lives and work?

Sit comfortably, taking nine deep breaths.

As you do so, open your imagination and vision to any images that come to you. It is okay if you feel a little light-headed.

Allow any visual images to arise. You can start with images from dreams, or you can listen for that still small voice.

The practice is looking and listening inwardly.

If you are distracted by thoughts, imagine they are choppy waves on the surface of the ocean and you can sink below them to a world of wonder and calm.

If nothing comes to you after some time, you can journey somewhere—anywhere you would like to go: the bottom of the ocean, high in the sky, on the beach, in the forest, on a mountain top, or even the moon. Trust what arises in you and go with the flow.

Corbin and Beautiful Painted Arrow tell us that there is a place of visions, so allow your active imagination to take you there. Allow the images to unfold, don't try to control them.

When you are ready to leave the place of visions, take nine deep breaths, gradually bringing your attention back into your body.

Feeling your fingers and toes.

Noticing how your breath connects you to the present moment in the place where you are now.

It can be helpful to jot down a few notes or to sketch out any images. This is what Jung did in *The Red Book*, creating a book of visions, like photos from a vacation to non-ordinary reality.

Just as meditation gets easier with practice, visioning gets easier with practice too. Jung recommended that you work with the images that arise and help to bring them into material form. This is where wording, drawing, painting, and all the expressive arts can be of service.

One of the most challenging things in visioning is allowing visions to arise and not stopping them or censoring them with the linear mind. There is a difference between making things up and allowing creative imagination to work through the visionary space you create for it. As images appear, begin to interact with them, treat them as visitors or guests. Even scary images can be worked with in this way, like the creature in my dream.

RECEIVING

> **receive** (v.) . . . from Latin *recipere* "regain, take back, bring back, carry back, recover; take to oneself, take in, admit"[243]

> *Becoming Medicine* means to be seeking healing, to be receiving healing, and then to be giving healing. *Seeking, finding/receiving,* and *giving* are the three fundamental stages of *becoming medicine* and these are three stages of initiation: *separation, initiation, return.*[244]
>
> DAVID KOPACZ AND JOSEPH RAEL

The work of receiving is more an emptying than a filling. If a bucket is full, you cannot put anything new into it. Joseph Rael often speaks of human beings as "medicine bags." What makes a bag useful is its emptiness. Burnout and soul loss can actually be helpful in this regard, as they can create the necessary space or emptying in order to receive something new and valuable.

As the etymology above suggests, *receiving* has a circularity about it; the prefix *re-* means to repeat, recover, recycle. Receiving is different than the ordinary, linear, logical reality. In *Becoming Medicine*, Joseph and I have a chapter on "Circle Medicine." As I was working with Joseph, learning about the circle of the medicine wheel (and in my work with veterans using the circle of the hero's and heroine's journey, and my work in Whole Health at the VA with the Circle of Health), I realized that holistic healing paradigms use a circular model, whereas clinical, evidence-based medicine uses a linear model. I was already familiar with the distinction between being a healer and a technician that I developed in *Re-humanizing Medicine,* and I now realized that being a healer meant working in holistic, circular, non-ordinary reality, whereas being a technician meant working in reductionistic, linear, ordinary reality.

Joseph often speaks of being a hollow bone that allows *Wah-Mah-Chi*, Breath-Matter-Movement, to flow through him, and that this is what being a healer is all about: getting out of the way and letting the Divine flow through. Here is how he puts it:

> Beautiful Painted Arrow is just a "hollow bone." I allow things to be done through me rather than doing things myself . . . Is Beautiful Painted Arrow a miracle worker? No, he is just a regular guy who eats chile and beans and whose wife tells him to eat healthy. He can't even speak proper English, but he likes to talk—talk, talk, talk.[245]

This quote highlights a distinction between identifying with the ego or identifying with the Self. Jung spoke of the path of individuation, the inner drive that rises up from the unconscious and directs the ego toward ever-expanding, greater wholeness. A psychology or philosophy that sees the contents of the ego (body, emotions, thoughts) as the totality of one's self blinds us to the transpersonal and inter-relational levels of the heart, creativity, intuition, and spirit. In *Caring for Self & Others*, we are speaking of the larger Self. Oftentimes the growth of the Self entails discomfort for the ego. While the ego generally seeks to accumulate things, emotions, and experiences, when the ego is working in service of the Self it must also focus on emptying, to create space for the Self to grow. Intuition is the ability to open oneself to the spiritual dimension. When the intuitive dimension fills with the spiritual, it overflows into the creative, and then you are bringing your vision into reality.

Joseph speaks of intentional suffering as a way of moving from ordinary to non-ordinary reality.[246] He describes the use of fasting, prolonged dancing, vision quest, and sweat lodge as ceremonies that break down the ego and create space for receiving Vast Self.

I have been lucky enough to participate in the Veteran's Sweat Lodge at the VA Puget Sound. Mike Lee, the ceremonial elder, leads veterans and staff through the *Inipi Olowan* (the Lakota word for the sweat lodge ceremony). One traditionally fasts that morning. Fasting breaks the usual routine of eating physical food in order to create emptiness for receiving spiritual food. You then sit in darkness as fragrant medicines (plants and herbs) are thrown on the glowing, hot stones. As you breathe in, the medicine inspires you. As you sit in the dark, you might see something through your inner eye of intuition, or maybe you are inspired to see something in your life differently. The heat from the stones brings you into the present moment and sharpens your mind, clearing out the clutter. It is a ceremony of purification that moves one from ordinary into non-ordinary reality. Once, during the ceremony, Mike said, "Everything is medicine because everything is sacred." When one is open to receiving the sacred in all things, then everything becomes medicine. "*Aho, mitakuye oyasin*," Mike often says during the ceremony, giving thanks to "all of our relations" on Mother Earth (as I spoke of in chapter 4).

The Human Heart as a Medicine Bag

> The human is a medicine bag. A medicine bag contains articles deemed sacred and holy by the person to whom the bag belongs. So it is with us. We carry holy "objects" in our psyche. The vibration of the sacred medicine bag is to see, to have capacities of the visionary. So, when we carry these forms, we carry the capacity of drinking the light, of being visionaries, exploring existence.[247]
>
> JOSEPH RAEL (BEAUTIFUL PAINTED ARROW)

In the realms of dreams and visions, we can receive sustaining and nourishing light. As Joseph often says, *to be a visionary is drinking light*. The human heart is an organ of transformation—transforming suffering into wisdom and compassion. Suffering can lead to breaking into a thousand pieces, yet suffering is also the raw material that we work with for transformation. The ancient Greeks recognized the dual nature of hurting and healing. The ancient Greek word for medicine was the same as the word for poison, *pharmakon*, and its effect depends upon how you use it.[248]

We can look at burnout as a kind of medicine that initiates a transformational process in our hearts. When we work with burnout, compassion fatigue, and soul loss—holding them within the medicine bag of our heart—suffering becomes medicine, poison becomes medicine. As *care-ers* for others, we take in the suffering of the world and we transform it into healing, giving healing back to others.

In the beginning, we think that medicine is out there, that it is something we need to obtain and something that has not happened yet. Joseph says,

> The thing I should have said in my books is that everyone already has their medicine. The way you become a medicine person is you practice who you are because you are already medicine. No one gives it to you, you are already it.[249]

RECEIVING PRACTICE—BECOMING A MEDICINE BAG

The work of the heart is to provide an empty space that is filled with blood and then emptied of blood. The heart is telling you that when you are doing heart-work, sometimes you will feel full and ful-filled, and other times you will feel empty, like you have nothing left to give. The problem is not the emptiness; the problem is the stress and tension that prevents you and your heart from relaxing into emptiness in order to become filled again.

Begin by sitting quietly, taking three deep breaths, and focus in on the four chambers of your heart.

Imagine your heart doing its heart-work: emptying, filling, emptying, filling, emptying, and filling. Allow your breath to find its rhythm as your heart does the heart-work of emptying and filling. Your breath is also emptying and filling. Your lungs fill with air as you breathe in. Your lungs empty as you breathe out.

A medicine bag is only useful if it is empty. It can only carry things if there is an empty space. Instead of focusing on trying to be full, instead embrace being empty. There is a theological term called ***kenosis***, which means a self-emptying in order to receive.

Rest in emptiness.

Rest in emptiness.

Rest in emptiness.

Allow yourself to be a "hollow bone." Embrace the emptying of your heart, the emptying of your mind, the emptying of your being.

Invite your imagination to show you what sacred and holy objects will fill the medicine bag of your heart. Allow your emptiness to receive the gift of healing. The gifts of healing are not yours to keep, rather they grow stronger through your capacity for giving them away, becoming even more empty in order that you may receive even greater gifts. Receiving is a gift, and the more you give away what you receive, the more you will receive.

Anchor the work by journaling, painting, drawing, or creating something that can remind you of the gifts that you carry within the medicine bag of your heart.

This may seem like an esoteric exercise, but it has a practical application for working with burnout, compassion fatigue, and soul loss—because these are states where we feel empty. Rather than trying to quickly cover over the feelings of emptiness, or going back to where we were, we can focus on going into the emptiness, allowing the emptiness to open us up. When our medicine bags are empty, we can then go on a visioning journey to the place of visions. Through intuiting, we can be led to where we need to go. In our emptiness we can be receiving the medicine that we need, which is the medicine we already have within us.

7

CARING FOR SPIRIT

Integrating—Unifying—Transforming

> Redefining who we are as human beings is a primary focus of the model of whole-person caring. Broadening our self-perception from biomedical entities to a perspective that acknowledges our spiritual nature is essential.[250]
>
> LUCIA THORNTON

SPIRIT IS THE place where everything is connected. We will explore three fundamental attributes of Caring for Spirit—*integrating* (different dimensions), *unifying* (within individuals, between individuals, and the global eco-community), and *transforming* (healing through unifying and integrating).

> **spirit** (n.) "… animating or vital principle in man and animals"… from Latin *spiritus* "a breathing (of respiration, also of the wind), breath; also "breath of a god," hence "inspiration; breath of life," hence life itself.[251]

Spirit, soul, vitality, breath, inspiration—these all are vital elements of what makes us human. Breathing brings inside and outside together in a harmonious balance. Two spiritual traditions exist: focusing on the spiritual as dwelling within (immanence) or the spiritual as being "out there, up there" (transcendence). Nondual mystical traditions combine both the immanent and the transcendent, seeing spirit as the essence of everything. The spiritual dimension is the place where paradoxes of both/and can stand side by side: you are a *unique individual*—and—you are also part of a *larger whole*. Spirituality is about becoming whole. The root of the word "whole" connects us to concepts of wholeness, holistic, holy, and healthy. All these words are related.

> **whole** (adj.) Old English *hal* "entire, whole; unhurt, uninjured, safe; healthy, sound;". . . from PIE **kailo-* "whole, uninjured, of good omen."[252]

David Tacey, a Jungian scholar from Australia, defines spirituality as including connection to self and the universe:

> We are forever trying to put things into formulas and rules. But I believe the seeking of the spiritual is a personal choice, and we cannot pin it down to any one tradition or code. It is best that we are not too prescriptive about it, and that our definitions are general and broad. For me, spirituality is not merely something we do when we are being self-consciously spiritual. It is the pursuit at all times—and not just in meditation or prayer times—of a particular attitude towards ourselves, the world and others. The attitude is one of reverence, awe, and openness to mystery. The spiritual attitude impels us to search for connectedness, and this search intensifies when we live in disconnected times such as now. There are many kinds of connection, but spiritual connection seeks relationship with something greater than ourselves, something that links us to the cosmos, but also to what is most genuine and true in ourselves.[253]

The VA Circle of Health includes a dimension called "Spirit & Soul: Growing & Connecting." Whenever I am teaching Whole Health to veterans or VA staff and introduce the Circle of Health, I define it as a feeling of vitality and connection to something larger than ego. I describe spirit and soul to clients as follows:

> "When we say spirit and soul, we are not necessarily talking about religion. Many people do find spirit and soul in religion, but we are talking about a universal human capacity to feel vital, alive, connected to something bigger than yourself. This could be an experience in nature, a peak experience playing sports, playing with your pets or kids, or any other experience in which you feel momentarily at peace and ease."

Similarly, in this chapter, I will speak at times about things that sound religious, but the original essence of religion was someone's experience of a *living spirituality*.

INTEGRATING

The evidence-base of Integrative Medicine has been growing and it is increasingly being incorporated into mainstream medicine. Complementary and Integrative Health (CIH) is an element of the Whole Health initiative at the VA. Similarly, meditation, mindfulness, yoga, guided imagery, tai chi, and other practices are becoming mainstream approaches for working with clinician wellness. While these modalities are being used in secular settings, they originated in various religious and spiritual traditions.

The influence of religion and spirituality on health has a growing literature and evidence-base.[254] The field of Integrative Medicine brings spirituality back into the practice of medicine, as spirituality is, itself, an integrating force. The spiritual brings disparate things together. For instance, look at the Earth—it has deserts, oceans, rainforests, mountains, valleys, caves, rivers, lakes, fields, rocks, glaciers, frozen places, and baked places. The Earth contains all these contradictory diversities, yet it is just one whole thing—the Earth. So, too, do you have many aspects of being: body, emotions, mind, heart, creativity, intuition, and spirituality. One of the functions of spirituality is to integrate these different dimensions into a complex and beautiful whole.

Think about what it means to be one-dimensional—one dimension is a point, like a period. If we say that a person is "one-dimensional," we mean he or she is limited in their understanding and interests. To be two-dimensional creates a line between two points. A piece of paper is almost only two-dimensional; it has height and width and then it has a very thin third dimension of thickness. Writing on a piece of paper is two-dimensional, which gives a more complex experience of reality than one dimension. The three-dimensional world of the body includes height, width, and depth. The three-dimensional world of the ego is body, emotions, and mind. A three-dimensional person has body, emotions, and mind.

We often limit ourselves to a three-dimensional reality, but the realm of the heart brings us into four-dimensional reality. Love transcends time and space, as sayings like "love knows no bounds" or "absence makes the heart grow fonder" point to. The love of the heart is an unseen quality that adds complexity and depth to the three-dimensional world of the ego. Love is a connection that transcends three-dimensional time and space. Similarly, using our dimensional model of human being, we could say creativity is the fifth dimension, intuition the sixth dimension, and spirit is the seventh dimension.

Each dimension is like a different language, or a different room in the "house" of your Self, or a different sound (like a vibration of a musical instrument). Each dimension is complete in and of itself, which can be isolated, studied, and perfected, yet it is an illusion to think that one dimension of human being exists without being linked to the other dimensions. We can develop each dimension, just as we can go to school to learn math, history, English, and science. Yet education is not just about math or just about history—education is about all fields of study and learning and none is more important than the others.

In the introduction I mentioned the philosophical concept of *antakolouthia*, where every virtue requires the others to complete it. This holistic concept brings together what seems separate into an integrated whole and is quite appropriate for our discussion of *caring for spirit*. In spirit, we are more than physical matter, more than emotional sensitivity, more than intellectual understanding, even more than love and compassion—we are whole, we are fully ourselves with each dimension integrated with the others, and with our Self integrating into the larger whole of humanity, global community/ecology, and the Universe.

Integrating the Human Dimensions

Various yoga traditions map out the universe of potential human experience on the body. The concept of chakras (*cakras* in Sanskrit) is that the energy or essence of each dimension maps on to a specific location in the body. The word "chakra" means "circle" or "wheel."[255] While chakras have been considered spiritual energy centers in yoga, Carl Jung described them as "symbols for human levels of consciousness," and the chakra system as "a symbolic theory of the psyche."[256] Thus, the chakras can be considered from a spiritual and a psychological perspective.

For our purposes, we can loosely consider the chakras and their map on the body as a way of doing a body scan that incorporates human dimensions, or levels of consciousness. In the following Human Scan exercise, you can incorporate the dimensions of the chakras or just follow the script. Different traditions have varying numbers of chakras used in meditation and spiritual practice. Seven chakra dimensions are commonly considered: the root chakra at the base of the pelvis (physical body), the emotional chakra between the navel and pelvic bone, the mental chakra between the navel and the rib cage, the heart chakra in the center of the chest, the throat chakra (creativity), the third eye at the center of the forehead (intuition), and the crown chakra at the top of the head (spirit). A variation of the Human Scan, as follows, would be to map the human dimensions on the body through the chakra system. The first seven dimensions of the ten dimensions of being fully human follow the chakra system and then add on space/context, time, and then coming full circle to leadership and caring for all.

INTEGRATING PRACTICE—HUMAN SCAN

This practice integrates the seven human dimensions we have covered thus far: body, emotions, mind, heart, creativity, intuition, and spirit. It can take some time to work through all seven dimensions. Don't feel like you need to do all seven at once; you can build up to them, doing as many as you like. You can also shorten the body scan to a quick tour through your body without stopping in various segments.

I invite you to find a comfortable seat or reclining posture and start by taking three breaths.

Bring your focus to your physical body.

You can do a brief body scan, bringing your attention to your face, your head, and your neck.

Then bring your focus to your shoulders, upper arms, lower arms, and hands.

Take a breath and feel your rib cage expand and contract as you breathe out, focusing on your torso.

Next, you can drop your attention down to your belly and low back, feeling your belly expand as you breathe in and contract as you breathe out.

When you are ready, shift your attention to your hips, pelvis, legs, knees, lower legs, ankles, and feet.

Take a few deep breaths here, enjoying the sensations of your body. If you'd like, you can move your whole body slowly and gently, either where you are sitting or standing, or lying on the floor. Now, let your body move you, let yourself be embodying. Remember, your body is made for moving. If you are moving, allow yourself to slowly find a comfortable position to resume your inner journey.

Next, invite your emotions in. They can be a bit messy at times, but don't worry about that. Just open the door and see who shows up. Take a few breaths and see if you can notice waves or the playing of different emotions.

When you are ready, bring your attention to your thoughts. Watch your thoughts go by like leaves floating on a river—coming and going, maybe swirling about. Sometimes your thoughts get caught on things, like sticks or rocks in the river. No worries, just watch the stream of consciousness do what it does.

Taking another deep breath, shift your focus to the center of your chest. Just as your lungs expand and contract with breathing, your heart is relaxing and opening up, and then contracting and closing down, creating a steady flow of oxygenated blood circulating throughout the body through the arteries and a steady flow of deoxygenated blood through your veins. Remember the Becoming a Medicine Bag practice, and the Loving-kindness practice. Just as your heart is circulating oxygen throughout your body, shift your focus to circulate loving-kindness within you, out into the world, and then back again inside you. Enjoy this feeling of the circulation of loving-kindness for as long as you would like.

When you are ready, bring your focus to your throat—the place where you speak out your words, the place of expression. If you'd like, you can put your palms on your throat and make a humming or buzzing sound. Feel the vibrations created in your throat. This is the place where you bring forth what is within you, mix it up in the world, and create your life. Observe the sensations in this part of your being, and notice if you feel any creative impulses yearning to come forth and be heard. Try giving voice to what lies dormant in your throat—speak, hum, or sing. Joseph Rael incorporates the five vowel sounds in his work, you can try this too—Ah (A), Eh (E), Eee (I), Ohh (O), Uuu (U).

The next dimension to visit is your intuition. Rub your hands vigorously and place both palms over your eyes for a time, feeling the warmth and darkness. Then rub them vigorously again and place one palm on your forehead. With your eyes closed, let your eyes wander, circling or shifting, looking internally in all directions. Open up to your intuition and see if any in-sights come to you. In dream sleep, your eyes enter Rapid Eye Movement (REM) sleep. You can simulate that by letting your eyes move themselves randomly and watching the play of colors, darkness, and movement. Unwind from the ever-present linear, forward focus of modern life and let your eyes relax back into your head.

When you are ready, bring your attention to the top of your head, your crown. Many cultures consider this part of your body to be sacred. You can imagine the fontanelle, the place where the bones of your skull fused when you were a child, to gently open or pulse. Imagine the insight of spirit coming to enter you. Regardless of any religious beliefs or affiliations, you can imagine inspiration entering through your crown and cascading down into all levels of your being.

Are you ready to do some integration work? After visiting each of these different dimensions of being fully human, you can now allow them to integrate so that they work together as a unit instead of as separate dimensions.

As you breathe, trace (in any color you wish) a line around your whole body. Then, in your imagination, allow this outline to be filled with waves of emotions, streams of thought, loving-kindness, the pulse of creation, the in-sights of intuition, and finally a sense of being vital and fully alive within as well as connected and engaged to all the world around you. Stay with this feeling as long as you like, allowing the integration of all seven dimensions of being fully human.

When you are finished, take three deep breaths, and slowly open your eyes. See if you can return to this experience of integration at other times throughout your daily life.

UNIFYING

The function of the ego is to create a separate identity of body, emotions, and mind. The heart, creativity, intuition, and spirit are sometimes called "transpersonal" dimensions. The transpersonal allows us to see that we are all related, we are all interconnected.

Spirit is about unifying, bringing together, seeing what is universal in all of us and in all things. We would not harm another person if we were truly in touch with our spiritual dimension, because we would recognize that in harming someone else, we are also harming ourselves and we are doing violence to spirit. Christian mystic Pierre Teilhard de Chardin writes, "Nothing is precious save what is yourself in others and others in yourself."[257]

As we spoke about Integrative Medicine in the previous section on integrating, here we will look at holistic medicine as a kind of *unifying medicine.*

> **holism** (n.) 1926, apparently coined by South African Gen. J.C. Smuts (1870–1950) in his book "Holism and Evolution" which treats evolution as a process of unification of separate parts; from Greek *holos* "whole" (from PIE root **sol-* "whole, well-kept") + -ism

> "This character of 'wholeness' meets us everywhere and points to something fundamental in the universe. Holism . . . is the term here coined for this fundamental factor operative towards the creation of wholes in the universe." [Smuts, *Holism and Evolution*, p.86][258]

Holism recognizes that everything is part of a larger *whole.* Vincent Di Stefano's book *Holism and Complementary Medicine: Origins and Principles* gives an excellent history of holistic medicine as well as describing its philosophy.

> Holistic medicine accepts that we are multidimensional beings whose health resides in more than the state of our biochemistry and organ systems. . . . Its essential aim is transformational; both practitioner and patient are changed in the process.[259]

A holistic and unifying way of experiencing Self and the world breaks down boundaries and the sense of separation. This can lead to mystical experience, the direct experience of a living spirituality. Every religion and spiritual tradition has a mystical branch in which the individual seeks a direct experience of God or spirit. Cultivating mystical experience is one way of recovering our souls, and the inspiration from mystical visions can motivate the transformation of individuals, practices, and cultures.

To have a mystical experience, you have to stop trying to be yourself so that you can be something else for a while. Maybe you become a tree, or a waterfall, or a sunset. These can be doors into mystical reality.

There are many different techniques, rituals, and ceremonies that can open us to a mystical experience. Dancing, singing, chanting, painting, meditating, doing yoga or tai chi, watching a candle or a campfire—all of these are activities where your sense of being a separate, isolated self can soften. This leads to a feeling of connecting to your true nature, connecting to others, to the Earth, even having a sense of reality in a different way. There is often a profound feeling of everything being okay just as it is. A mystical experience is a flow state in which you have an experience of nonduality and interconnection. Mysticism is the experience of unifying.

Interspirituality: a Civilization with Heart

Joseph Rael is fond of saying he is a *cosmic citizen* and that we should all aspire to cosmic citizenship. This is similar to Brother Wayne Teasdale's concepts of interspirituality and intermysticism, movements that bring us together as citizens of the Earth. Teasdale sees these trends as "preparing the way for a universal civilization: a civilization with a heart."[260]

Teasdale describes nine elements of interspirituality:

1. Spiritual practice
2. Simplicity of life
3. Mature self-knowledge
4. Humility
5. Solidarity with all living beings
6. Actual moral capacity
7. Deep nonviolence
8. Selfless service and compassionate action
9. Prophetic voice[261]

We can apply these elements of interspirituality to our work as health care workers, educators, and leaders. In these roles we take on a moral responsibility for the well-being and growth of those in our care. The ideal of selfless service and compassionate action can actually be an interspiritual practice. Interspirituality grows out of the unifying, mystical sense of our interconnection with life. When we feel interconnected, we realize that we are responsible for more than the happenings within our ego.

Spirituality is part of being fully human, and if we are going to *re-humanize medicine*, we also need to *re-spiritualize medicine* as well. Without spirit, we are de-spirited and we experience soul loss. Without inspiration, we only have expiration. Teasdale sees interspirituality as a transformative force for individuals and society:

> Spirituality . . . is an essential resource of transformation of consciousness on our planet, and it will be enormously beneficial in our attempts to build a universal society . . . I believe there is a real possibility for a genuine renaissance of the sacred, and with its dawning comes the hope of a universal civilization with a compassionate, loving heart. If that compassionate, loving heart is cultivated in a large number of people, then the universal age will be born. It all depends on . . . intermysticism that is open to all.[262]

Regardless of your religious beliefs, the spiritual dimension can help us to feel whole again after burnout, compassion fatigue, and soul loss. The challenge is for us to practice and cultivate interspirituality so that we can work together to create a health care and educational culture with a heart.

Mysticism & Medicine

I had a section in *Re-humanizing Medicine* on "Mysticism, Medicine, and the Perception of Reality." While mysticism might seem esoteric to some, it has an ancient tradition linked to healing. There is a practical dimension of mysticism because if we change our perception, we are able to transform who we are. Mystics of world traditions speak of reaching a place where the boundaries between self and other fall away.

> [A] high understanding it is, inwardly to see and know that God, which is our maker, dwelleth in our soul; and an higher understanding it is inwardly to see and to know that our soul, that is made, dwelleth in God's substance: of which substance God, we are that we are.[263]
>
> DAME JULIAN OF NORWICH

One of the hallmarks of mysticism is experiencing a state of oneness with all of creation. To become a mystic, one must cultivate mystical experiences. These may come through intuitive practices, such as opening and receiving. As Joseph Rael reminds us, the microcosm is the macrocosm, the heart of the medicine wheel is your heart, the heart of the Earth, the heart of the Universe, and it is even the Heart of God—*Wah-Mah-Chi*. As I have mentioned before, *Wah-Mah-Chi* is the Tiwa language word for God and also translates into English as "breath-matter-movement." These are three separate words or concepts, but when you put them together, you get an entirely new concept that integrates the three elements into a larger whole. Joseph would also say that God is in breath, in matter, and in movement, so the divine is both immanent and transcendent.

In *Becoming Medicine*, Joseph and I wrote about the cave of the heart and developed a ceremony or practice for exploring this inner spiritual landscape. In Hinduism, the cave of the heart is known as *guhā*, and Teasdale gives the following description:

> The rishic seers, the mystic founders of Hinduism, also experienced continuity between the divine presence encompassing the entire cosmos and the inner depths of their own hearts, the *guha* or cave of the heart, the deepest point of human subjectivity and freedom, a 'place' uncorrupted by time and external actions. In India, the *guha* is a metaphor for that hidden, transcendent place within us that is totally transparent to the divine . . .

> the deepest center of ourselves is one with the deepest center of the universe.[264]

Mystical experiences break down the boundaries between self and other, human and nature, and human and divine. I would like to take the idea of mysticism and medicine even further in this book, developing a kind of medicine that emerges from Oneness.

Nondual Medicine

The radical materialist paradigm views everything and everyone as separated objects, like a universe of billiard balls colliding yet remaining separate. It can be difficult to connect and care across this gap between the self and other. If we experience ourselves as not separate—as nondual, not two, non-different—then to care for self is to care for other and to care for other is to care for self. This is *nondual medicine.*

Larry Dossey is a former Vietnam War combat surgeon and current leader in exploring science and healing, and a proponent of what I am calling nondual medicine. In his book *Reinventing Medicine,* he describes three eras of medicine: Era I (physical medicine), Era II (mind-body medicine), and Era III (nonlocal medicine). "Nonlocal" means that we interconnect and interact with each other through nonphysical ways. Dossey states that "nonlocal medicine does not confine or localize the mind to the brain and body," and further that "the mind is *more* than the brain."[265] He discusses the implications of nonlocal medicine in regard to the Golden Rule:

> Do unto others as you would have them do unto you. . . . We can see that the Golden Rule takes a thoroughly local point of view. That is, it assumes we are separate entities—I am I, you are you, and we are doing things to each other. But [nonlocal medicine] recognizes the collective, unbounded nature of human consciousness. It maintains that while our bodies may be separate, our minds are not. In [nonlocal medicine], "I" and "other" are in some sense one, which means that what we do to others we do to

> ourselves. This makes possible an extension of the Golden Rule: "Do good unto others because they *are* you![266]

While Dossey draws on ancient spiritual traditions for nonlocal medicine, he also reviews the science in *Reinventing Medicine* and in his later book, *One Mind: How Our Individual Mind Is Part of a Greater Consciousness and Why It Matters*. The concept of the One Mind, Dossey writes, "is a collective, unitary domain of intelligence, of which all individual minds are a part."[267] I won't go into Dossey's review of the science necessary to support this paradigm shift, you can examine that yourself if you wish. For now, let's entertain the implications of Dossey's conclusion.

> Each of us has broken our responsibilities to our earth and environment, therefore to ourselves and to one another . . . Yet it is within our power to redeem our shortcomings by reclaiming nonlocal nature—the One Mind that unites us all with all else, including our earth; the One Mind whose calling card is love, caring, affection. When we sense our place in the Great Connect, our response is to honor that with which we are linked, as if it were our lover.[268]

Dossey's concept of One Mind and nonlocal medicine is a kind of nondualism in which separation between self and other evaporates. I would now like to offer the idea of *nondual medicine* for consideration as we work to care for self while caring for others.

I have mentioned my work with Joseph Rael and his koan-like statement that "we do not exist." I have also mentioned my certification training in iRest (Integrative Restoration), which Richard Miller developed based on elements of yoga nidra. Consider Miller's definition:

> Yoga Nidra is a process of self-inquiry, that entails disidentification from the content of consciousness and deconstruction of the mind's core belief that it is a separate ego-I. Disidentification and deconstruction heal the misperception of separation and brings an end to

> suffering. Disidentification constitutes our capacity to experience life without reactive defense, releasing us from the myth of separation and revealing our True Nature as nondual Presence.[269]

Nondualism is a difficult topic to comprehend because it is beyond intellectual comprehension, but rather a state of being beyond thought and concept. Don't worry if it doesn't make sense to you—every time I have tried to follow Joseph Rael down the rabbit hole of "we don't exist," it does my head in—which I imagine is actually the point! What I hope to introduce with the concept of nondual medicine is that it is possible to cultivate a spiritual experience of nonduality in which self and other are not separate, which has profound implications for burnout, compassion fatigue, and soul loss, as they are states of separation from self and other. Nondual medicine connects us into a kind of power current that is the essence of spiritual reality, in which the flow of caring and love is reality. And now back to our regularly scheduled programming . . .

UNIFYING PRACTICE— BEAUTIFUL PAINTED ARROW ON SOUL RECOVERY

"Here is my contribution for working with Burnout and Soul Loss:

I did a lot of work on burnout and soul loss. I trained in hypnosis.

If you are doing soul work, you have to imagine that at this time, on planet Earth, we are separated by a river, the River of No Return. When you cross to one side to the other, you have communities on both parts. We are all separated, you know, we have the right and the left hemispheres of our brains. We are separated but still we are one. Indians call it the River of No Return. It is called that because there were two lovers from two different pueblos whose people wouldn't let them marry and they jumped in the river and they drowned.

In order to handle burnout, when you get tired you lie down and use hypnosis, like I do. Part of you is on the left side of the river and part of you is on the right side of the river. What you need to do is to jump in the river, do it fast because there is a current.

You jump in and you swim from the right to the left and then you climb out and get the part of you that is over there and then you jump back in and you swim from left to right and get the part of you that is over there. You do it individually for clearing fatigue. You have to do it in the water because the water kills the flame of burnout. Swimming across is like making a bridge to connect the two sides.

If you are working with patients, or another person, have them do it physically. Have them lie down and imagine swimming back and forth across the river. If you are going to be in contact with patients every day, you have to bring your right side to your left side—you jump off this drop, down into the river and there is a splash as you drop into the water, then you have to go swimming together. When you get to the other side you run out to the one person on the left, then you jump back in and swim over to the person on the right. Then you are back whole.

You've spent 20 minutes or maybe not even that. Make it a thing you do every night. That's the way I found to stay out of the trouble with burnout and soul loss." [270]

JOSEPH RAEL (BEAUTIFUL PAINTED ARROW)

TRANSFORMING

The secret of change is to focus all of your energy not on fighting the old, but on building the new.[271]

DAN MILLMAN

Transforming means more than just changing what you do; it entails changing who you are. We are constantly transitioning in our lives.

Every 120 days, we make new blood cells, and our body is continually converting the food we eat into our very bodies. We transition through life stages, moving from infancy to childhood, childhood to adulthood. We graduate, we get jobs, we start relationships and end relationships, we get married or divorced, have kids (or not), retire, and eventually pass on from this world. Traditional societies had elders who helped structure these transformational transitions with rituals and ceremonies. Without guidance through transformation and transition, we can become lost and disoriented.

Sociologist Jack Mezirow studied transformative learning and found that it begins with disorientation, similar to the process of initiation. Transformative learning begins with a "disorienting dilemma," which leads to recognition of "a connection between one's discontent and the process of transformation," and finally there is a return, a "reintegration into one's life on the basis of conditions dictated by one's new perspective."[272] This model of transformative learning is not just changing what we do (learning new facts or techniques), but entails a transformation of who we are. Transformative learning has been compared to the Jungian concept of individuation, where learning "is transformation—emergence of the self."[273] Mezirow saw that disorientation and confusion are necessary for transformation. Can we see our burnout, our compassion fatigue, and our soul loss as the first step of a disorienting dilemma that leads to transformation of ourselves and our institutions?

Initiation & Transformation of the Soul

Michael Meade has written a marvelous book called *Awakening the Soul: A Deep Response to a Troubled World.* Meade tells us that it is just when things seem most hopeless that the resources of the soul are most mobilized for transformation of ourselves and the world. Crisis is an opportunity for initiation and transformation. He tells us that the human soul is "the underlying and unifying force of life," and that it carries "an inheritance of resiliency and a capacity for innovation in the face of disaster."[274] This resiliency is what we are looking for when we are working on transforming burnout, compassion fatigue, and soul loss.

> As the inner dynamic of transformation, initiation means the continuous breaking open of areas of the soul to reveal hidden capacities and inherent gifts. When life pulls at us from the outside and the soul pushes us from the inside, we reach the point where pain and longing requires that we change. . . . Whatever interrupts, breaks us open, or breaks us down—whether it is the trauma and shock of a loss in life or the drama and exhilaration of success—also initiates us into a greater knowledge of ourselves.[275]

Meade tells us, just like Mezirow, that times of disorientation are invitations to the initiation of transformation. The soul is this agent of transformation. When we are working in the realm of spirit and soul, we are also unifying and integrating all levels and dimensions. Thus, the work of transformation of the individual soul is also the work of transforming the collective, world soul. At the level of spirit and soul, microcosm and macrocosm are unified and transformational healing is distributed throughout life systems. As Meade writes,

> Transformation at the level of the individual soul generates the imagination and collective energy needed to change the conditions of the world. What we need is not a minor repair, but a major transformation of the world that can only start from the inside. The true path for changing and healing the world lies in the awakening of the individual soul.[276]

While burnout and compassion fatigue can feel like we have lost our souls, it is not so much our souls that are lost as we who are lost—we have lost touch with the innermost being of ourselves. As Joseph Rael teaches, *Wah-Mah-Chi*, Breath-Matter-Movement, holds back a place of goodness in each of our hearts, no matter what we have done and no matter what has been done to us. Burnout and compassion fatigue can be viewed as *disorienting dilemmas* that start the initiation of transformative learning—post-burnout growth! In this way, periodically losing touch with ourselves (our souls) is actually an ongoing invitation to enter into the healing space of transformational initiation. Our troubles, disorienting as they are, can be the call of transformation. "Thus," writes Meade, "the troubles we find ourselves in are intended to wake us up to a greater sense of life and awaken the underlying soul, which knows better than us what our life is for."[277] The loss of energy in burnout and compassion fatigue creates a space that offers us the opportunity to be guided by our inner knowing and inner wisdom of the soul. For, as Meade tells us, "when our energy drains from life's outer projects, our attention is drawn inward, downward and back towards the original spark of our lives and the genuine project of our soul."[278]

Becoming a Liminal Being: Living in Transformation

In *Becoming Medicine*, Joseph and I wrote about the concept of liminal beings—inbetweeners who spend time between different roles and places. "Liminal" comes from the Latin *limen*, meaning "threshold." For instance, subliminal means "below the threshold." The idea of liminality is popular amongst those who study change, as it can be seen as the in-between state, or gateway, between the old and the new. Anthropologist Victor Turner wrote about the process of initiation, which he described as having three stages: "separation, margin (or *limen*...), and aggregation."

> The attributes of liminality or of liminal *personae* ("threshold people") are necessarily ambiguous, since this condition and these persons elude or slip through the network of classifications that normally locate states and positions in cultural space. Liminal entities are neither here nor there; they are betwixt and between the positions assigned and arrayed by law, custom, convention.... Thus, liminality is frequently likened to death, being in a womb, to invisibility, to darkness.... It as though they are being reduced or ground down to a uniform condition to be fashioned anew and endowed with additional powers to enable them to cope with their new station in life.[279]

Liminality sounds a lot like burnout, compassion fatigue, and soul loss. Who would want to feel this way—*reduced or ground down*, like *death*, *invisibility*, or being lost in the *dark*? A person of transformation—that is who! As health care workers, we put ourselves into the liminal space between life and death, between health and illness, and between suffering and well-being.

After working in primary care mental health integration for some time, I realized that I was supposed to feel tension because my job was to be a bridge and a shock absorber between two different systems that thought in two different ways: mental health and primary care. I realized that I was an *inbetweener*, a *threshold person*, a *liminal being*. As a liminal psychiatrist, I try to remind myself that my job is to experience the tension between systems and also to stay in this in-between place with the client. Psychologist Eduardo Duran says the difference between a psychologist and a shaman is that psychologists "take the patient all the way to the edge of the cliff and leave him there," whereas a shaman will "push him over the cliff and go with him, and stay with him as long as it takes to bring him back."[280] This resembles what I have been learning about healing from Joseph Rael, that the shaman's scope of practice is moving between worlds and being a liminal being. Rather than trying to fit clients into boxes, I try to meet them where they are between boxes and between worlds. This also means being present with pain and suffering—others' as well as my own. While the liminal space can be disorienting, it is where all the good stuff is, and it is where transformation happens.

The Transformation of Things

Taoists speak of the "transformation of things" as an inner force of continual transformation within all life. Caring for Spirit asks us to make peace with continual transformation and to become comfortable not knowing who we are and being in between. Here is a passage from Chuang Tzu (also known as Chuang Chou), a 4th century BCE Chinese philosopher and sage:

> Once Chuang Chou dreamt he was a butterfly, a butterfly flitting and fluttering around, happy with himself and doing as he pleased. He didn't know he was Chuang Chou.

> Suddenly he woke up and there he was, solid and unmistakable Chuang Chou. But he didn't know if he was Chuang Chou who had dreamt he was a butterfly, or a butterfly dreaming he was Chuang Chou. Between Chuang Chou and a butterfly there must be *some* distinction! This is called the Transformation of Things.[281]

TRANSFORMING PRACTICE—TREE OF LIFE

Find a comfortable pose and close your eyes and take a few deep breaths.

Imagine yourself as an acorn.

Imagine a squirrel buried you in the ground in the autumn and forgot about you. Now it is spring and the cold snow begins to melt. You are planted into the ground, buried in darkness, then flooded with water. You are soggy, cold, and in the dark—yet something stirs inside you.

You split open and a sprout root starts to grow downward in the soil (remember, you always have to go down before you can go up).

Then you start to grow upward, pushing through the soil, up into the light, and your first leaves unfurl. Half of you is in darkness reaching downward, absorbing nutrients and water from the soil. Half of you is in the light, the chlorophyll in your leaves absorbing sunlight, absorbing carbon dioxide, and giving off oxygen. You cannot be a sprout in the sun without having your roots buried in the darkness of the soil.

Transforming from acorn to a sprout might be disorienting, it might even be painful, but it is a movement toward a larger purpose as you go through the liminal space from underground to above ground.

Now, imagine years of growth from a sprout . . . to a sapling . . . to a small tree . . . a medium-sized tree . . . and eventually a full-grown tree in full maturity. Is this you? Is this who you have been struggling to become—a tall, beautiful, strong, and sturdy oak tree?

Time continues. You lose branches, your upward growth stops, but you continue to gain in character, in uniqueness, as you keep on growing in different ways. Birds nest in your branches and squirrels make a home in a hollow in your trunk. You create a crop of acorns every year.

Maybe one of the squirrels living in a hole in your trunk is the great, great, great grandchild of the squirrel who buried you in the ground oh so many years ago. Maybe one of these great, great, great grandchildren buries one of your acorns in the ground one autumn and forgets to dig it up. When spring comes, one of your acorns sprouts, going through the same early stages of growth that you went through. Maybe this sprout is trying to grow, but your branches are shading the little sapling.

There is a meaning and purpose to what looks like your breakdown and decay. Having created new life, you must become the fertilizer for it and create a space for the upcoming generation to occupy and come to full fruition. This is the circle of life, receiving the life you are given, then giving life away—this is the way of transformation.

Eventually you pass away and pass on yourself, but you have lived in the world, you have struggled to grow and become who you are—not just a frozen moment of youth, but a complex and multi-faceted being: growing, transforming over time. Just like the seed or acorn, we begin in the Earth and we return to it. Your life has come full circle. This is what is known as the Transformation of Things.

8

CARING FOR CONTEXT

Harmonizing—Sustaining—Communing

> As caring professionals, we cannot undertake any professional activity without consideration of the context of the world in which we find ourselves. It is important to situate ourselves and our professional work within the larger issues of the world, particularly with regard to environmental concerns.[282]
>
> SALLY ATKINS AND MELIA SNYDER

CONTEXT IS MORE than the backdrop within which we live our individual lives; it is part of a dynamic interaction between what shapes us and what we shape in our lives. Context includes your physical, human-made environment, your relationships, and your surroundings, as well as the natural world. We will explore three fundamental attributes of Caring for Context—*harmonizing* (being in balance), *sustaining* (caring for our home ecosystem), and *communing* (the process of attunement between inner and outer environments). We will look at how our relationship with context can either cause or heal burnout, compassion fatigue, and soul loss. In looking at our larger context, we must also look to the health of our environment and ecosystem, which also is suffering from eco-burnout.

Context shapes us, yet we also shape our context—this statement is an example of holistic systems thinking, which physicist Fritjof Capra and chemist Pier Luigi Luisi describe as "complex . . . nonlinear . . . networks," with "countless interconnections between the biological, cognitive, social, and ecological dimensions of life."[283] On one level, we appear to be separate beings, but we are also inseparable from the larger whole. Capra and Luisi write that the "material world, ultimately, is a network of inseparable patterns of relationships . . . the planet as a whole is a living, self-regulating system."[284]

HARMONIZING

> **harmony** (n.) . . . from Greek *harmonia* "agreement, concord of sounds". . . literally "means of joining," used of ship-planks, etc., also "settled government, order," related to *harmos* "fastenings of a door; shoulder," from PIE . . . **ar-* "to fit together"[285]

To harmonize is to be in relationship, to be in agreement, to fit together in a coordinated way. This means that within the individual, there is balance between dimensions, and externally, there is harmony with people and the environment. When we "click" with someone, we say, "We are on the same wavelength," but when we don't click, we might say, "I just don't resonate with them."

Harmonizing brings together the various inner parts of the human being as well as all the outer people and beings in our environment. The ancients spoke of health as being a balance of inner and outer, microcosm and macrocosm, Heaven (above) and Earth (below). Pythagoras spoke of the harmony of the spheres, the hidden singing of the planets and stars. Taoist sages described health as the balance of yin and yang, masculine and feminine, and being in harmony with the Tao.

> Lao Tzu said: As heaven reaches its heights and earth reaches its depths, as sun and moon shine, as the stars

> twinkle, as yin and yang harmonize, there is no contrivance in any of this. Make the way right, and things will spontaneously be natural.
>
> It is not yin and yang and the four seasons that give birth to the myriad of things; it is not timely showers of rain and dew that nurture the plants and trees; when the spirits are connected and yin and yang harmonize, the myriad beings are born.[286]
>
> *WEN-TZU*, VERSE 11

In Western culture, medicine seeks to break us down into smaller and smaller component parts, focusing solely on chemical reactions and not larger-scale relationships. This is why Joseph Rael and I have introduced the harmonizing concept of circle medicine.

> Rather than separating or reducing a person into separate organs, circular medicine seeks to bring the person together into wholeness and to look at how to re-orient or harmonize a person with reality—with self, with other people, with community, and with nature. "*Life is a Being and we are all parts of that Being*," Joseph tells me.[287]

We are in relationship with everything. We are connected to everything. Life itself is based on balance and equilibrium, what scientists call *homeostasis* (maintaining a constant internal environment while in relation to the external environment). As the environment around us is constantly changing, so too must we constantly change and adapt.

In her book *Healing Spaces: The Science of Place and Well-Being*, Dr. Esther Sternberg writes that the "idea that physical space might contribute to healing, does, it turns out, have a scientific basis."[288] She cites Ulrich's classic study that found patients whose hospital rooms had an external window healed more rapidly than those who had no window.[289] Sternberg points out that in the pre-scientific era, people knew that health and well-being were linked to harmonizing with the environment. For instance, the Greek healing temples of Asclepius were built "far from the heat, noise, dirt, and dust from towns, always at freshwater sources, usually with a magnificent view of the sea," where patients were treated "with healthy diet, pure water, music, sleep and dreams, social interactions, and above all prayer."[290] Throughout history, people have sought out nature and the arts to create a context for recovering from illness, building resilience, and creating well-being.

Harmonic Resonance

Biologist and biophysicist James Oschman has written about the Schumann resonance, electromagnetic waves that oscillate at an average frequency of 7–10 Hz between the surface of the Earth and the ionosphere. He points out that the Schumann resonance overlaps with the alpha rhythms of the brain, which have been found to increase during states of meditation. He describes the concept of "entrainment," where two rhythms become harmonized with each other—for instance, the brain waves of a meditating person and the Schumann waves in the atmosphere. Thus, the benefit of meditation could be that we literally entrain to the Schumann resonance and get back in harmony with the Earth.

Oschman further reviewed research findings that showed that the brains of healers from different spiritual traditions not only entered into the characteristic alpha rhythm of a meditative state, but these rhythms also "became phase and frequency synchronized with the earth's geoelectric micropulsations—the Schumann resonance."[291]

The implication of these findings is that when we meditate or shift into deep healing states, we harmonize with the vibratory frequency of the Earth. In our daily lives, we get busy and we run on frequencies of time, pressure, and productivity. But when we pause, breathe, meditate, and focus on healing, we are naturally drawn back through harmonic resonance and entrainment with the vibration of the Earth. Recall the discussion of the studies from HeartMath that showed that two people's hearts (EKG) and brains (EEG) can entrain and harmonize with each other when sitting together. Perhaps this is how healing works—that a healer enters into a meditative healing state, harmonizes their heart and brain waves with the Schumann frequency of Mother Earth, and then sends this frequency of loving-kindness to the person needing healing. Harmonizing truly could be the underlying basis of healing!

Śavāsana & Incubation

It is common practice in a yoga class to end with the *śavāsana* pose, the pose of the corpse. After all the work and exertion during the class, the final pose is a rest pose, lying flat on the Earth, not striving for anything, but simply being. Perhaps at this time we entrain to the Schumann resonance of the Earth. *Śavāsana* is similar to an ancient Greek practice from the healing temples of Asclepius (Asklepios) called incubation. Psychotherapist Edward Tick describes incubation in his book *Soul Medicine: Healing through Dream Incubation, Visions, Oracles, and Pilgrimage.* Tick describes incubation as "temple sleep," in which the "seeker fasted, prayed, meditated, and waited, until they received a 'big dream' or vision."[292] Incubation was a process of letting go of the ego, the conscious mind, ceasing striving, and opening up to create space for a healing vision that would re-harmonize the individual with the divine.

Peter Kingsley has also studied and practiced the ancient Greek healing ritual of incubation. Peter is a friend of Joseph Rael's, and he and I have spoken over the years I have worked with Joseph. His work links the ancient Greek healers to the contemporary work of Carl Jung and Henry Corbin. Here is how he describes incubation.

> What's important is that you would do absolutely nothing. The point came when you wouldn't struggle or make an effort. You'd just have to surrender to your condition. You would lie down as if you were dead; wait without eating or moving, sometimes for days at a time. And you'd wait for the healing to come from somewhere else, from another level of awareness and another level of being.[293]

HARMONIZING PRACTICE—RESONATING WITH YOUR ENVIRONMENT

Sit or lie down in a quiet place. Find a comfortable posture. Take three deep breaths.

Listen to the sounds around you, whatever sounds they are—birds, traffic, appliances—and attune yourself to them.

See if you can harmonize with them. Try softly humming in frequency with whatever sounds are around you. Try focusing in on different sounds and mirroring them with your humming. Notice how you feel with different vibrations. Even if you find the sounds unsettling, they are always there in your environment; try for a bit to harmonize with them before you make any changes in your environment or move to a different location.

Next, see if you can allow all the human-made sounds to fade into the background. Feel or imagine the Schumann resonance of the Earth, the vibratory pulsations of the living ecosystem all around you. This vibration is always there in the background, all you need to do is to breathe, pause, and let yourself attune to and harmonize with the rhythm of the Earth.

If you'd like, lie down and practice śavāsana, the pose of the corpse, allowing your ego to silence in order to make space for healing to visit you. Or maybe you'd like to try incubation; find some dark and quiet place and curl up and wait for a healing visitation in a dream, an image, or a vision.

Harmonizing is based on sympathetic resonance and bringing heart, mind, spirit, and environment into vibratory alignment. As you go about your day, notice the effect your environment has on your well-being. For instance, listen to the sounds arising from pouring a cup of coffee, tea, or water. See if you can hear the musical notes going up the scale as the liquid nears the rim. What else do you hear? Listen. Can you hear/feel the quiet but persistent pulsations of the Earth?

SUSTAINING

No matter how many patients you've seen in a day, there is always one more waiting for you at home—you, and your self-care and well-being regimen that is needed in order for you to return to work to be efficient and productive the next day. It doesn't seem fair that institutional medicine can burn you out, then blame you for feeling used up, and assign you the task of engaging in superhuman and heroic self-care in order to be able to return to work so that you can be used up again and again. The way we are working is not sustainable.

Schwartz, Gomes, and McCarthy have declared that "The way we're working isn't working." They further point out that "the relentless urgency that characterizes most corporate cultures undermines creativity, engagement, thoughtful deliberation, and, ultimately, performance," with a "series of silent costs: less capacity for focused attention, less time for any given task, and less opportunity to think reflectively and long term."[294]

Many doctors and health care workers are expressing concern about the unsustainability of health care work environments. Dr. Danielle Ofri's article "The Business of Health Care Depends on Exploiting Doctors and Nurses" makes the argument that institutions exploit the compassion and caring of health care workers' professionalism to boost productivity:

> Increasingly, though, I've come to the uncomfortable realization that this ethic [of compassionate professionalism] that I hold so dear is being cynically manipulated. By now, corporate medicine has milked just about all the "efficiency" it can out of the system. With mergers and streamlining, it has pushed the productivity numbers about as far as they can go. But one resource that seems endless—and free—is the professional ethic of medical staff members.[295]

Physician Victor Montori calls for "a revolution of care" to transform the context of our work environments. "My goal," he writes, "is to persuade you that we must transform healthcare from an industrial activity into a deeply human one, capable of providing careful and kind care for all."[296] This is like my idea of the compassion revolution, that we need to transform health care so that we can actually take the time to care. How can we transform our work environments so that care is valued and prioritized?

Sustaining Work Environments

When we talk about caring for context with burnout, let's consider the impact of the system on the individual. We need to somehow create contexts of caring in our work environments. Just as nature is an ecosystem of many interconnected parts, so too are our work environments—complex ecosystems with a multitude of interwoven elements.

Maslach and Leiter have introduced the analogy of the canary in the coal mine for burnout, which is a very ecological example. It encourages us to shift from focusing solely on the canary (the individual health care worker) and to look at the contextual toxins and stressors in the work environment. Maslach and Leiter remind us of the fundamental attribution error, "the tendency to focus on figures versus ground, and to cast other humans as figures," which leads to more "dispositional judgments than situational ones."[297] A dispositional judgment reduces the complexity of outcomes to blaming individual personality or characteristics, rather than taking into consideration the context of the situation. This is a reduction from ecosystem to individual, or ignoring the "ground" and only focusing on the "figure." It is not the canary's fault that the mine is toxic, and building more resilient canaries is not a sustaining, ecological, systems-based solution. As the authors state:

> The bottom line on burnout is that it is a social phenomenon, not an individual weakness. Interpersonal and organizational solutions need to be framed in terms of "we" and "us"—a sociocentric view rather than the "I" and "me" of an egocentric one—and they need to be shared and reciprocated by everyone . . . When the relationship between workers and their workplace is functioning well, then the former will thrive, and the latter will succeed—truly a win-win situation.[298]

If we are caring for context, we need to all work together to create contexts of caring which are sustaining for workers as well as economically sustainable. Work environments need to be designed around human needs, not industrial, institutional needs. We will pick up this theme again in chapter 10 with the section on Leading Caring.

Sustaining: Being in the Service of Life

We hear a lot about sustainability in relation to human life and our relationship with the natural world. When something is not sustainable, we are taking more out of the environment than can be maintained long-term. Examples are shrinking forests from logging, depleted fish populations in the ocean, and putting more and more carbon into the atmosphere. Sustaining—to live in a sustainable way—is a function of the relationship of the inner and the outer, of the individual and society, and of society and the environment.

Capra and Luisi state that "a sustainable society must be designed in such a way that its ways of life, business, economy, physical structures, and technologies do not interfere with nature's inherent ability to sustain life."[299] Sustaining reminds us that we are working in the service of others and the service of life.

We talk about sustainable agriculture (meaning farming practices that give back to the land rather than short-term hyper-production, which causes long-term problems) and sustainable economies (that value long-term viability over short-term profits). Sustainability means thinking long-term. In many Indigenous cultures, this means thinking beyond your own lifetime to how your decisions impact the next seven generations.

> We are the International Council of Thirteen Indigenous Grandmothers. We have united as one. Ours is an alliance of prayer, education, and healing for our Mother Earth—for all Her inhabitants, for all the children, and for the next seven generations.[300]

Beautiful Painted Arrow made a similar appeal in his 2009 "Message to the Elders," which was the closing for his book *Sound*.

> As elders we have more responsibility . . . a responsibility to talk about the sacredness of the Earth, and the sacredness of the people of the Earth. One of our journeys is to help people as they walk on Mother Earth. Mother Earth is our land and she belongs to us because we are her children.

> She belongs to us and we belong to her. So we can take care of her the way she has been taking care of us.[301]

If we were thinking of the next seven generations, we would have been more mindful about the creation of so much plastic, which can take hundreds of years to decompose.[302] Plastics are found in just about everything—clothes, electronics, furniture, buildings, cars, toys, packing materials, envelopes, and medical equipment. Plastics are inexpensive in the short term, but the problem is that they resist decomposition when no longer in use. Scientists are finding all sizes of plastics in the ocean, which are getting into our food chain and from there are getting into me and you as microplastics.[303] The thoughtless and indiscriminate use of plastics is not sustainable because we are contaminating our environment with them and also using fossil fuels to make them.

Nuclear energy is another practice that is not sustainable if we take into consideration the long-term costs. The half-life of plutonium is 24,000 years and our plans for managing this ever-growing amount of radioactive waste are for considerably shorter periods of time.[304] In the United States and many Western societies, our economy is based on a philosophy of ever-increasing growth, ever-increasing profits, and the production of an endless stream of new gadgets without considering whether short-term gains are sustainable long-term. We prioritize economy over ecosystem.

The climate crisis is another result of unsustainable living. Psychiatrist Robert Jay Lifton writes that climate change "confronts us with the most demanding and unique psychological task ever faced by humankind," reminding us that it is not just a technological problem, but a psychological and political problem as well.[305]

Sustaining Earth Medicine

In their book *Sustaining Life: How Human Health Depends on Biodiversity*, physicians Chivian and Bernstein have put together a call to action to protect the species of the Earth. We are in such a dire situation of risking a "sixth great extinction event" because "our behavior is the result of a basic failure to recognize that human beings are an inseparable part of Nature and that we cannot damage it without severely damaging ourselves."[306] This book inspires us with the natural beauty of the Earth, warns us about the unsustainable path we are on, and provides practical things that everyone can do to sustain our civilization and the Earth.

Over the past few years, I have become increasingly interested in the concept of medical activism (which will be discussed in more detail in chapter 10), because we face so many environmental, public health, and political health issues. I think of medical activism as the practice of medicine or health care when it goes beyond the four walls of the clinic consultation room. For instance, climate change is now being recognized by health professionals as a public health crisis,[307] and in 2021, over 200 medical and science journals around the world published a call to action.[308]

All the problems in society and the climate crisis can be demoralizing. But what can we do as individual doctors, clinicians, and health care workers? Here are some ideas:

- Develop a professional identity as a healer and moral agent, not only a technician and protocol manager.
- Write, educate.
- Shift your identity from that of an isolated individual to part of a web of interconnected beings, viewing everything in the world as your relations.
- Cultivate nondualism—where there are no "others," only Self.
- Make wise choices with your life and purchases.
- Educate yourself about the health benefits of plants and gardening and encourage patients to work with plants as part of their treatment plan.[309]
- Plant ten trees (in your yard, or through services for off-setting your carbon footprint).

- Convert 30% of your lawn to native plants—what Douglas Tallamy calls Homegrown National Park.[310]

- Plant native plant species[311] or plants that support butterflies and bees.[312]

- Stop using leaf blowers (these waste energy to blow your "waste"—potential compost and habitat for beneficial insects—into other people's yards, and also create air and noise pollution).

- Put together a conference—we did! Along with several other groups, The Doctor as a Humanist put on the Nature & Medicine Symposium in November 2021.[313]

While much of climate awareness has to do with what we need to stop doing, I also like to focus on the things that we can do to support biodiversity and to create healthy natural environments. You can start in your own backyard. We can become everyday naturalists through regular harmonizing with nature.[314] Rather than looking at the climate as a problem we need to solve, we can focus on sustaining a healthy relationship with Mother Earth.

Climate Neurosis

In certain depth psychotherapies, the goal is to make the unconscious conscious. The theory is that mental illness is caused by a lack of harmony or a clash between our conscious attitude and our unconscious reality—in other words, neurosis. The treatment is to make friends with the unconscious and expand consciousness.

There are a number of names for the syndrome of distress about the environment: climate despair, eco-anxiety, climate anxiety, ecological grief, solastalgia, eco-angst, environmental distress, and ecological trauma.[315] These are the symptoms and syndromes of climate neurosis.

Maybe these symptoms and syndromes are not really pathological, perhaps they are signs of being sane and in touch with reality in an insane culture. If we shift from looking at the individual to looking at cultures, a cultural/environmental problem could be viewed as a cultural neurosis. This is a misalignment between cultural consciousness and the truth and reality of the unconscious. With our current environmental crisis, we could consider this a cultural climate neurosis—our conscious way of living is in conflict with the unconscious reality which is the truth of the natural world.

Treating climate neurosis would then require us, as individuals and as a culture, to make the unconscious conscious—to learn about the truth of the natural world and how we can better harmonize and create sustaining relationships. Treating climate neurosis also requires us to expand our mode of consciousness. One way of doing this is to expand our view of consciousness, extending the identity of consciousness and personhood to animals and plants, and even to the way different ecosystems are alive and purposeful and seek homeostasis. We can consider the Earth herself to be a conscious person, which is why Joseph Rael is always speaking of Mother Earth. To treat climate neurosis, we need to change our relationships so that they are more sustaining.

Sustaining Hope

Before we can take action to make the world a better place and to create a more sustainable society, we first need to sustain hope—otherwise we despair, we get demoralized, and we give up. For my New Year's resolution in 2022, I decided to read a book a month on hope. As with many of the topics in this book, hope is something that requires a continual practice in order to renew and sustain our sense of it. A few of the books I read include *The Book of Hope: A Survival Guide for Trying Times* by Jane Goodall and Douglas Abrams; *Active Hope: How to Face the Mess We're in without Going Crazy* by Joanna Macy and Chris Johnstone; *Hope in the Dark: Untold Histories, Wild Possibilities* and *Orwell's Roses* by Rebecca Solnit; *Zen and the Art of Saving the Planet* by Thich Nhat Hanh; and *Sacred Earth, Sacred Soul: Celtic Wisdom for Reawakening to What Our Souls Know and Healing the World* by John Philip Newell.

I have found this immersion in books on hope to be a kind of practice, a practice of hope. As with any sustained practice, there is a deepening benefit over time. Practices are helpful for cultivating values or mindsets that easily get put on the backburner due to the distractions of everyday life. The practice of hope builds and sustains hope. Hope is a renewable resource, something that we must find within ourselves before we can work to make a more hopeful world.

Burnout, compassion fatigue, and soul loss are all about the loss of hope as well as the loss of vitality. In these states, we can come to feel that nothing matters, that nothing we do makes a difference, that no matter how hard we try things will get worse. What happens when we think of burnout, compassion fatigue, and soul loss in the context of health care, education, politics, and the environment? One answer to these overwhelming dilemmas is the cultivation of hope. In a way, the heart of this whole book is in restoring hope once it has been lost, and then restoring hope for others. We need to care enough to hope.

SUSTAINING PRACTICE—A PERSONAL ECOLOGICAL STUDY

> **ecology (n.)** *oecology*, "branch of science dealing with the relationship of living things to their environments," coined . . . by German zoologist Ernst Haeckel as *Ökologie*, from Greek *oikos* "house, dwelling place, habitation". . . + -*logia* "study of"[316]

The word *oikos* is Greek for "home," and the word "ecology" thus means the study of home. To study your home is a kind of ecological study.

Find a comfortable posture. Take three deep breaths.

Look around at the objects that surround you. Where do these come from? How often do you use them? Where do they go when you are done with them? How sustainable is your life?

In your journal or on a piece of paper, jot down some observations about the sustainability of your home environment. Write down some action points for different ways you can live your life and make your choices on purchases and discarding things with an eye to creating more sustainability.

As part of this practice, you can study what you throw away for a week. This is what archaeologists do to learn about a culture—they study the material remains of the culture. You can study your own household culture for a week.

As you study your material culture in the garbage that you throw away, notice each piece of rubbish—is it a natural element that will decompose? Is it human-made? How long will it take to decompose? Is it recyclable? Do you know for sure? There is a term called "aspirational recycling," where you put something in recycling hoping that it can be recycled, but really you are just complicating the recycling process by trying to recycle what cannot be recycled. Also, are you aware of the limits of plastic recycling? Plastics can only be recycled two or three times before the polymer chains break down and it is then trash that goes into the environment.[317]

It can feel daunting to face the question of sustainability, but if we do not become conscious of how our daily lifestyles are or are not sustaining ourselves, others, and the Earth, then we will be unconsciously contributing to the problem. We all need to enter into treatment for our individual climate neurosis, which makes up our collective climate neurosis.

It is normal if this practice makes you demoralized, but remember, this pain and distress is not yours alone to bear; it is part of our common ecological psychotherapy that we must all do together as a culture.

If you feel like you need some hope, you can add this sustaining practice.

Find a comfortable posture.

Take a few deep breaths. Notice how your breath sustains your body. Notice the wisdom of your breath and how it works with your environment, exchanging oxygen and carbon dioxide.

Find a plant—either in your house, out your window, or even in a crack in the sidewalk. It doesn't have to be a special plant;

> it could be a blade of grass or a scraggly weed. With your in-breath, imagine oxygen released from the plant coming into your body, where you use the oxygen and transform it into carbon dioxide. On your out-breath, imagine carbon dioxide leaving your body and being absorbed by the plant and converted to oxygen again. Settle into a gentle rhythm of the plant providing what you need, sustaining you, and you providing what the plant needs, sustaining it. This is the essence of sustaining and sustainability. Observe this cycle of sustainability for as long as you wish.

Nature is inherently based on sustaining relationships. Although our society and our individual lives can be out of balance and out of harmony, we can turn to the natural world and be taught all we need to know about the principle of sustaining from even the most modest leaf of grass. In his poem "Song of Myself" from his book *Leaves of Grass*, Walt Whitman meditates on the glories of our shared atoms and the inherently sustaining nature of reality. Whitman made his book *Leaves of Grass* into a practice, revising it and editing it throughout his life, resulting in multiple different versions. While a simple leaf of grass can teach us the wisdom of sustaining, a sustaining practice requires a lifetime of harmonizing and re-harmonizing to support.

COMMUNING

Communing is a form of relationship with our context. We commune with other people to form relationship, and ultimately, community. We also commune with nature and relate to animals and our earthly environment. Both these types of communing are integral in order to care for self & others and can help us reignite the flame of our healer's heart and soul.

Pathologies of Context: Individual, Social, Political, and Moral

The health impacts of sedentary lifestyles, as well as abundant fast food and other aspects of Western life, have been described as "affluenza"—the health impacts that come from over-abundance.[318] A dark parallel to affluenza is what Case and Deaton describe as "deaths of despair," when they noticed that life expectancies have been going down in segments of the population within the United States. They describe these deaths of despair as being related to pain, addiction, alcoholism, and suicide.[319] Quinones describes the cultural shifts happening within US culture that have led to the opiate epidemic, which significantly overlaps with deaths of despair.[320] Wilkinson and Pickett, in their book *The Spirit Level*, describe how growing inequalities in societies are leading to poorer health outcomes for everyone, rich and poor alike. As with the concept of affluenza, the authors describe how the "successes" of industrial societies negatively affect the health of everyone.

> It is a remarkable paradox that, at the pinnacle of human material and technical achievement, we find ourselves anxiety-ridden, prone to depression, worried about how others see us, unsure of our friendships, driven to consume and with little or no community life. Lacking the relaxed social comfort and emotional satisfaction we all need, we seek comfort in over-eating, obsessive shopping, and spending, or become prey to excessive alcohol, psychoactive medications and illegal drugs.
>
> How is it that we have created so much mental and emotional suffering despite levels of wealth and comfort unprecedented in human history? . . . We talk as if our lives were a constant battle for psychological survival, struggling against stress and emotional exhaustion, but the truth is that the luxury and extravagance of our lives is so great that it threatens the planet.[321]

The suffering that Wilkinson and Pickett describe sounds a lot like the burnout that people are feeling in their jobs. Perhaps part of what we are feeling in health care is not just about our professions, but about our larger culture. Our context affects our bodies, minds, health, and spirits. Cultural values around work ethic, our mistreatment of the environment, and the selfishness of a *me first* attitude have real health impacts. It can be overwhelming to face all of these social issues, which have come to be called the social determinants of health. Many researchers hold that these social ills arise from our sense of separation from others and our sense of self that includes only self and not others.

Don Berwick, former president of the Institute for Healthcare Improvement and former administrator of the Centers for Medicare and Medicaid Services, calls on us to start viewing the social determinants of health as the "moral determinants of health."

> Healers are called to heal. When the fabric of communities upon which health depends is torn, then healers are called to mend it. The moral law within insists so. Improving the social determinants of health will be brought at last to a boil only by the heat of the moral determinants of health.[322]

Berwick is pointing out the inseparability of individual and community health. When the fabric of the community is unwell, then individuals will be unwell. Berwick bears witness to health inequalities and inequities and moves us from a passive description of the social determinants of health into an active engagement with the moral determinants of health. This is the essence of medical activism, giving us a moral imperative to attend to issues outside of the clinic that impact the health of individuals and communities. This informs a public health philosophy where the health of one affects the health of all.

Context connects our bodies with each other through our culture. Historical and intergenerational trauma persist within our culture and our political bodies, as van der Kolk reminds us of how the individual body keeps the score of insults from trauma. Resmaa Menakem writes of racialized trauma that is embodied within all our bodies, regardless of skin color, and that the health of each of us, and the health of our culture and society, depends upon us all healing our nervous systems and bodies.[323] He offers a number of mind-body exercises for this work.

Rhonda V. Magee also calls for a mind-body approach in her book *The Inner Work of Racial Justice*. She describes how through personal mindfulness practices "we can begin to ground and heal, and ultimately transform our sense of self, no longer clinging too tightly to a narrow and isolated sense of 'I,' 'me,' 'my wounds,' and the collective pain-stories of 'my people.'"[324] Just as mindfulness can help us face the difficult waters of our inner suffering as individuals, Magee tells us that mindfulness can help heal our outer suffering in society by making us more resilient—resilient in social justice as well as resilient as an individual. "Justice," she writes, "begins with our awareness of the present moment, extends through caring for ourselves, and shows up in the love we bring to our interactions with others and our responses to the social challenges of our time."[325] What we could call mindful justice awareness allows us "to reconnect what has been artificially separated and to maintain those connections throughout our days . . . We seek, in other words, a deep and revolutionary mindfulness with the capacity to awaken us to our role in the suffering of others and support us in enacting transformative justice."[326]

We can view pain, discomfort, burnout, and the moral determinants of health as signs, as communications that something is not right in our individual bodies, or within our body politic. Social and racial justice issues contribute to burnout, moral injury, and soul loss. Doing the work of sustaining and communing can seem overwhelming these days. There are so many problems and so many issues—and these problems will not go away by ignoring them. Just as we as individuals must work to re-ignite our souls, so too must we work as society to address the health of us all.

There is a lot of work going on focusing on diversity, equity, and inclusion (DEI), ranging from individual to systemic levels. Some of this DEI work includes training to avoid micro-aggressions. While this is important work, healing society will require more than stopping causing more pain. We also need to cultivate micro-compassions, for ourselves as well as others. Just as many small aggressions can have a larger negative impact, we must not forget that many small compassions can have a larger positive impact. We do not do the work of caring for self & others because it is easy, or because we will succeed. We care for self & others because to not care is to lose our humanity.

This is what Martin Luther King Jr. called creating the Beloved Community, as I mentioned in chapter 4. "The aftermath of nonviolence,"

Dr. King said, "is the creation of the beloved community, while the aftermath of violence is tragic bitterness."[327] The question of how to create this Beloved Community through nonviolence is as much a medical issue as it is a social, political, and moral issue. We are all in communion with each other. Dr. King said:

> It really boils down to this: that all life is interrelated. We are all caught in an inescapable network of mutuality, tied into a single garment of destiny. Whatever affects one directly, affects all indirectly. We are made to live together because of the interrelated structure of reality.[328]

Communing with Others

To commune with someone is to be in a deepening relationship. It is a practice of being open, a kind of loving-kindness practice in community. Throughout history, people have developed communes—gatherings of like-minded people who come together in a special place with a common goal and vision. Can we bring an aspect of the commune into our daily work—where we commune with each other?

We've discussed the concept of *communitas* earlier in the book and it is worth revisiting as we discuss communing. Victor and Edith Turner were a husband and wife anthropologist team who developed the concept of *communitas* to describe the breakdown of normal social boundaries, which then allowed for the flourishing of fully human-to-human relationships. Edith Turner wrote that "The communitas element is present in religious healing wherever there is human contact between a healer and sufferer. *Communitas* is the general term for love, community, fellow feeling, compassion, sympathy, and the search for the benefit and response of another soul."[329] *Communitas*, the breaking down of boundaries between individuals, is present in healing, as well as functioning as a source of healing our painful divisions. The Turners initially studied *communitas* in non-industrialized societies, but also traced its outbreak historically throughout the world, as well as finding it in movements like the 1960's counter-culture. Edith Turner further describes *communitas*:

> The benefits of communitas are joy, healing, mutual help, collective religious experience, long-term ties with others, a humanistic conscience, and the human rights ideal. . . . The implications follow that if one responds to communitas, one can no longer treat another human being as an object, because each soul is too much part of other people's souls. . . . We exist in a vast interchange of spirit personality—often glimpsed, sometimes seen clearly in the acts of spirit sociality. The social itself can become a matter of intuitions passed between people and a joyous sense of bonding, sometimes providing the power of collective healing and of acting in visionary harmony.[330]

We come together for a common purpose and with a common vision. This brings in concepts of whole health, including all aspects of health and well-being. The busy-ness and protocols that we work with can interfere with the true business of our work—healing the whole self of clients. Sometimes we have to set aside schedules, service lines, data entry, and computerized checklists, and connect with a patient's experience of pain and disharmony. It can be challenging to find the time to have a chat with a colleague, take a walk, get lunch or a coffee, but when we do this kind of social and communal action, we might find a little bit of *communitas*, feeling less isolated and having a degree of a feeling of oneness.

Communing with Nature

> Rootedness is a way of being in concert with the wilderness—and wildness—that sustains humans and all life. The rooted pathways offered here are not meant as a definitive list but as waymarkers and fortification for all of us seeking our unique, bewildering, awkward way through the essential question of how to live on our broken, imperiled beloved earth.[331]
>
> LYANDA LYNN HAUPT

Throughout history, humans have turned to nature for rejuvenation and wisdom. "The art of healing is rooted in nature," Dr. Carl von Essen reminds us, and humankind "has treated illness and injury for thousands of centuries with plants and minerals that have often yielded remarkable results."[332] We are drawn to nature for healing, for well-being, and for relaxation. Biologist Edward O. Wilson writes about *biophilia* (literally the love of life), which he defines as "the innately emotional affiliation of human beings to other living organisms."[333] There is a connection between living things that goes beyond what can be stated in words.

Charles Foster's fascinating book *Being a Beast: Adventures Across the Species Divide*, describes his experiences in deep communion with various animals by trying to live as much like them as possible in the wild. He digs a badger den, eats worms, tries to catch a fish in the river with his mouth and hands, and gets hassled by the police for hanging out in a city park trying to commune with foxes.

> I want to know what it is like to be a wild thing. . . . This book is an attempt to see the world from the height of naked Welsh badgers, London foxes, Exmoor otters, Oxford swifts, and Scottish and West County red deer . . . It's a sort of literary shamanism, and it has been fantastic fun.[334]

Foster used two methods for communing; first he would read the relevant literature, and then he would immerse himself in the animal's world, for instance living underground like a badger for six weeks. He really put himself in the animal's worldview as much as possible. With a wry sense of humor, he says that a person who talks to their dog "is acknowledging the porosity of the boundary between species" and has "taken the first and most important step toward becoming a shaman."[335] His book is a meditation on what it is to be a human animal as compared to a regular animal.

> What's an animal? It's a rolling conversation with the land from which it comes and of which it consists. What's a human? It's a rolling conversation with the land from which it comes and of which it consists—but more stilted, stammering conversation than that of most wild animals.[336]

COMMUNING PRACTICE— CONNECTING WITH YOUR RELATIONS

Foster writes that "You get good relationships by relating."[337] Similarly you will get good at *communitas* and community by communing. You don't have to go to the lengths that Foster did, living underground for six weeks, but you do have to get at least a little out of your comfort zone. You can do this practice with a person, a pet, by getting out in nature in your backyard or a park, or in Nature with a capital "N," somewhere "out there." Realize, however, that you are part of nature, even sitting in a room reading this book at this moment. There is nowhere you can go that you are not part of nature. There is nothing on Earth (other than some meteorites and whatever is in Area 51) that did not come from the Earth. Even "man-made" materials are still made of Earth.

Begin by finding a comfortable seat or posture.

Close your eyes and take three deep breaths.

Listen to the sounds around you, smell the scents, feel the air on your skin, and touch whatever is nearby you. Notice how these other senses become more alive when you aren't processing visual information.

Open your eyes with a soft focus and look around at your environment.

When your eyes find something of interest that you would like to commune with, imagine that your boundaries are becoming more porous. You can call this subject your communing partner.

Enter into a silent conversation with your communing partner. See if you can imagine some kind of information exchange, some kind of contact between yourself and your communing partner. For instance, if it is a tree, see if you can feel into what it is like to be a tree. Similarly, do so for a flower, a dog, a cat, a bird, a person, a park bench, your wooden bookshelf, or even a cloud or the sun or moon. It may seem like you are imagining it, but let yourself partake in the being of this being.

You may want to let this communing subject know that you are going to do a practice for a minute, but you'll be back. Now imagine yourself having very tight, firm, strong boundaries. Pull your imagination back within the boundary of your body and look at your communing subject, and see if there is a difference in your relationship. What does it feel like to be withdrawn into yourself compared to communing with another? You can do this back and forth, opening and closing your boundaries. Let your boundaries relax again, entering back into communion for as long as you like.

When you are finished, thank your communing partner. Take three deep breaths, and continue on with your day. See if you can remember to practice communing with others throughout your day. When we feel connected to someone, it is easier to practice caring.

9

CARING FOR TIME

Growing—Transitioning—Becoming

> My further desire in planning this book was to create a narrative that would engage the reader intent on discovering a trajectory in her or his own life, a coherent and meaningful story, at a time in our cultural and biological history when it has become an attractive option to lose faith in the meaning of our lives. At a time when many see little more on the horizon but the suggestion of a dark future.[338]
>
> BARRY LOPEZ

WE ARE OFTEN hurrying in our work environments—are we missing the suffering around us even if we have good intentions? There is a study that tells us about how time pressure can interfere with caring. The study's subjects read a short passage on the Good Samaritan. Then some subjects were told they had ample time to get across campus and give a short talk on the Good Samaritan, while other subjects were told they had just enough time, and the last group was told to hurry because they were late. A shabbily dressed member of the research team was lying on the ground near where the subjects had to walk. Of those study subjects in the "high hurry" sample, only 10% stopped to help, whereas 63% in the "low hurry" group offered assistance.[339] This is important for us to remember, because if we think we can multi-task, or if we are rushing between meetings or patients, we can miss another's suffering. Compassion takes time.

We move through time and unfold and grow in our lives. While we exist only in this present moment, it is also true that we come from a place and we are growing toward another place. We will explore three attributes of Caring for Time—*growing* (unfolding through new experiences), *transitioning* (moving between different life stages) and *becoming who you are* (bringing our inner truth into relationship with the world).

It is a fundamental reality that we are transitory beings—we are in transit through time. It is a fundamental paradox in our identities that as we move through time, we both remain who we are and yet we are continually growing and changing. We have both a tendency to try to resist change, staying as we are, and also a tendency to embrace change and become who we could be.

Einstein is famous for the theory of relativity, which explores how time is experienced differently depending upon how fast you are moving. Have you experienced periods in your life where time seemed to move more quickly or slowly? Think about how when you are "in the zone" or in a flow state, that time can both stretch out and become more spacious, so that even hard work passes smoothly and effortlessly. Sometimes in a flow state, time moves more quickly; you think you've been doing something for a few minutes while an hour passed on the clock. In contrast, think about other periods in your life where time seemed interminable and torturous. You might have been counting down the minutes before some anticipated event, or until some long and arduous task was completed. What is it that makes time move fast or slowly from a subjective perspective?

The time pressures of contemporary health care, education, and leadership contribute to our burnout, compassion fatigue, and soul loss. However, when we enter deeply into caring, our experience of time can change. Jean Watson has written extensively on caring and describes the transpersonal caring moment as extending beyond individual boundaries and also transcending time, space, and separation. Watson has found that when we enter into caring, time and space expand.

> Transpersonal caring is considered metaphysical in that the entire consciousness of caring and love exists within a single caring moment; that moment transcends time, space, and physicality. Transpersonal also indicates that a new field of connection with infinity is possible in that moment—beyond ego . . . participants are fully embodied, immanent, and transcendent in the present "now."[340]

Caring for self & others takes time. If we take that time, we can grow and transition in the never-ending process of becoming who we are.

GROWING

> When knowledge asks new questions, space itself expands. In this more spacious realm, time slows down. In this new time frame, mind can operate differently.[341]
>
> TARTHANG TULKU

As we move through time, we are continually having new experiences: we are developing, learning, changing, adapting, and evolving. We start as a spark and combination of genes from our mother and father, we are born, we grow through childhood, teenage years, young adulthood, middle age, and old age. It is like a ride at the amusement park and our bodies are the cart that we ride in, with our personality learning and growing as it goes on the ride.

As the pre-Socratic Greek philosopher Heraclitus said, "All things change."[342] The truth of life is that we are always growing. Just when you think you have it figured out, it seems like the rules change and you have to adjust and adapt.

But just how does that change occur? In what ways do you resist change? How can we embrace change to become change experts and less of change resisters?

> **grow** (v.) Old English *growan* (of plants) "to flourish, increase, develop, get bigger". . . from Proto-Germanic **gro-* . . . from PIE root **ghre-* "to grow, become green"[343]

The word "grow" has its roots in the growing of vegetation and becoming green. Hildegard of Bingen, known as one of the Doctors of the Church, wrote of *viriditas*, which is sometimes translated as "greening." Mirabai Starr writes that Hildegard "coined the term viriditas to evoke the lush, extravagant, moist, and verdant quality of the Divine, manifesting as 'the greening power' that permeates all that is."[344]

How are we *greening* and *growing* our lives? We can study nature for the natural process of growing, and we can seek to find that within ourselves that wishes to grow, like the blind force of a seed, buried in the cold, dark ground that knows how to reach the light.

GROWING PRACTICE—HEALING WOUNDS

In our physical bodies, we grow throughout our lives. Just as we are growing physically, we are also growing in all the human dimensions of body, emotions, mind, heart, creativity, intuition, and spirit, plus time and context. It is our experience of time that makes growth possible. Without time, we would have stagnation. In this practice, we will first focus on how the physical body heals from a wound, which is a type of growth. Next, choose a non-physical wound which you might be working with or struggling with in your life.

Please find a comfortable place and posture.

Notice your breath moving in and out of your lungs and your lungs expanding and contracting with each breath.

Notice your belly's movement with each breath as your diaphragm is contracting and relaxing.

Recall or imagine when you had a small cut in your skin. Maybe you cared for the cut yourself or maybe someone else cared for your wound.

Imagine cleaning out the cut, putting some antibiotic ointment on it, putting on a bandage.

In your imagination, enter into the wound itself. Imagine how all the cells of your skin, your blood, and immune system work together to stop the bleeding, prevent infection, and begin to heal the wound.

Consider the four stages of wound healing: 1) hemostasis (where your blood clotting system is activated), 2) inflammation (where redness and swelling occur), 3) proliferation (where tissue cells begin to grow and close the wound), and 4) tissue remodeling (where scab and scar revision occurs).

Trust that your body knows how to heal when it is given time to work. It is not something you have to try to do; healing is something you are. Each of us has this inner healer who is always growing, healing, remodeling.

If you would like, you can try a second part of this practice. Imagine a non-physical wound—something emotional, mental, in your heart, soul, or spirit. For instance, a broken heart, a hole in your soul, or a darkened spirit.

Imagine how this wound you are working with might be visually represented. For instance, with a broken heart, first it shatters into pieces, then you try to put the pieces back together but the swelling prevents it. Then your heart starts to heal and repair, but there may still be pain as your heart cells proliferate and then remodel.

Or maybe you feel like you've been stabbed in the back. First, you need to take out the knife, and there will be some blood flow, but then your clotting system kicks in. There is painful swelling and tenderness for some time. You might feel as if the wound is closed, but there is a scab that feels vulnerable to getting knocked off. Finally, you might feel that your wound has remodeled and has now healed.

Picture what it would look like for this wound representation to go through the stages of healing. How would the blood flow stop? What would it feel like to have inflammation, redness, and swelling after the wound, and how would that gradually subside?

How would the edges of the wound be brought together through the proliferation of cells? How would the wound be remodeled and revised to minimize scarring?

If you can collect the pieces of your wound, clean them and bring them together, then hold them patiently, your body knows how to heal. Healing is an innate potential we all have within us. Our work is to support the healing medicine within ourselves.

After doing this practice in your imagination, journal for a bit, or do some creative work putting the images into physical form through drawing, painting, or some other activity.

TRANSITIONING

Akin to the idea of growing is the concept of transitioning. Transitioning represents the movement from one phase to another. As we move through life, we go through many predictable phases and steps. You can think of these as life steps or passages. Gail Sheehy wrote *Passages: Predictable Crises of Adult Life* drawing on the earlier lifespan developmental work of Daniel Levinson's *The Seasons of a Man's Life* and Erik Erickson's *Identity and the Life Cycle*. Midlife (or "midlife crisis") is another transition that many have written about, such as Murray Stein's *In Midlife: A Jungian Perspective* and Arthur C. Brooks' *From Strength to Strength: Finding Success, Happiness, and Deep Purpose in the Second Half of Life*. These books focus on life's transitions and challenges that we face at different times in our lives. Although we are individuals, we all pass through similar challenges from birth, childhood, teenage years, young adulthood, middle age, old age, and death.

We all move through transitions. Sometimes transitions are smooth and other times they are rocky and tumultuous. Transitioning can be thought of as a death and re-birth. We reach the pinnacle of our development, say as a child, and then we move into teenage years and suddenly face a whole different set of challenges. We have to "die" to our old identity as a child who is taken care of to grow into a new identity as a being of self-responsibility. Similarly, at mid-life, the self of the first half of life often doesn't seem to work as well. In an often-painful process, it dies, and a new self is born out of the ashes. Although Jung didn't coin the term "mid-life crisis," he wrote a great deal about the mid-life transition as part of his process of individuation—the drive for wholeness—that was a centerpiece of his work.

Apocalypse as Liminality

Remember in chapter 7, Caring for Spirit, in the section on transforming, we reviewed the concept of liminality—the state of being between, being an *inbetweener*. To embrace liminality is to embrace transitioning in life. Sometimes the rate of change or the magnitude of change can feel like an apocalypse, like with the COVID-19 pandemic—a dramatic destruction of our life as we know it. Much of the pain and fear around change is that we are thrust into liminality; we've lost the old way but haven't yet developed the new, thus we are caught between two worlds.

Michael Meade tells us that if we follow the word *apocalypse* back to its roots, we find "ancient Greek terms like *apokalein* and *apokalypsis*… [which] mean 'to reveal' and 'to uncover;' they can also mean 'to disclose' and 'to discover.'"[345] Apocalypse, according to Meade, is as much about lifting the veil and discovering something new as it is about the destruction of what we have known. Our fear of apocalypse, which is really our fear of change, can paralyze us and blind us to possibilities. An antidote is to see that our soul is at home in the liminal space between the old and the new, as Meade tells us, that the "human soul is a betwixt and between thing."[346]

Burnout, compassion fatigue, and soul loss can feel like an apocalypse. Honor, acknowledge, and sit with that. In an interview I did with him, Richard Miller described thinking of burnout as a messenger.

> That's the terminology I've introduced into iRest, which is burnout is a messenger, we're not trying to get rid of it. We are bringing it in for dialogue and inquiry: "What brings you here into my life? What do I need to learn from you, so that I can become so sensitive to you that as in the future, I move towards you?" I'm recognizing you more early on as a symptom and a messenger that is

> telling me I need to shift something, so that I don't go all the way into the burnout.[347]

Meade counsels that the burnout and fatigue that put us in the place of soul loss can also be an invitation and initiation into encountering our souls in the *liminal betwixt and between*. According to Meade, the soul is found in crisis and disorientation.

> For the great crises of the world do not take place outside the human soul; history is made through the struggle of the soul to survive and make meaning of the world around it. The inner-seeded story of the individual soul is secretly tied to the great drama of the world and to the surprising ways in which it changes, renews, and recreates itself. Acknowledgment of what has been lost and acceptance of feelings of exile are not symptoms to be treated as much as a requirement for finding genuine ways to proceed. . . . The issue is not simply one of needing to save the world, but also of needing to solve the problem of the loss of the soul throughout the modern world.[348]

Mark Epstein, a psychiatrist who integrates Buddhist wisdom into his work, teaches us that "pain is not pathology" and by "creating an inner environment of attunement and responsiveness, even the most unendurable and crushing reality" can become "not only bearable but illuminating."[349] If we can face our fears of change and apocalypse and enter into the liminal space of betwixt and between, we can encounter our lost souls and reignite the flame of the heart of the healer.

Healing ourselves and healing the world turns out to be part of the same process. We are all working to create a caring home for ourselves and others. Michael Meade writes of how it is just when we feel lost that we are closest to being found:

> Everyone at some point finds themselves in the ashes of life and longs for home. The real home turns out to be the center within each life and each return to that inner core

not only calms us, heals us and makes us whole, but also adds some healing and wholeness to the world around us. When the end seems near, it becomes time to seek the center within and find ways to be central to the healing of the scorched and scarred earth around us. The great tragedies and dramas of life and the threat of it all ending try to return humanity to an awareness of the eternal presence of the divine waiting at the center of each life and all life.[350]

TRANSITIONING PRACTICE— THE CREATIVE PULSATION IN THE APOCALYPSE

We often think that life is meant to be stable and happily ever after, but life is in the spaces in between. Just as Joseph Rael says that "God is in the spaces, not in the words,"[351] it is in the spaces that we live our lives. It is in the spaces that Matter can Breathe and Move, giving us *Wah-Mah-Chi*, Breath-Matter-Movement, the Tiwa word for God.

Psychotherapist Dina Glouberman has explored the opportunities that burnout can provide in her book *The Joy of Burnout*. She writes that joy "emerges in the spaces rather than in the content of our lives."[352] If we shift from focusing on objects and materialism to focusing on the movement and continual growth and transitions in life, we cling less to the past. There is a Sufi saying that "we need to die before we die,"[353] encouraging us to let go into what we are in the process of becoming. Becoming a liminal being means that you make friends with the process of letting go so that you can step into joy, and maybe even *Wah-Mah-Chi*, or God, in the spaces of your life.

I invite you to close your eyes and find a meditative space.

Settle into the usual way that you experience your self—contained within your body and mind.

Picture something in your immediate environment and experience, looking from the perspective of a subject perceiving an object.

Now imagine a field of energy that has two poles, the object and yourself. Imagine the energy in the space between you and the object. Now see if you can experience being the interconnecting space between you and the object. Take a deep breath into this space.

Next, imagine your consciousness as something not bounded by your brain or body, but as a moving energy and force that continually pulses between your body and the object. Relax into this—maybe it is a wave moving back and forth, like radio frequency waves, or like a flickering fire, or a vibration, or a light, or colored lights. Sink into this feeling of living movement, pulsing and flickering between yourself and the object.

In the Kashmiri Shaivism branch of Hinduism there is the principle of *spanda*, "creative pulsation, divine activity, throbbing with life, dynamism."[354] See if you can feel yourself as a vibration of consciousness. See if you can feel all of existence as pulsating vibration. Allow yourself to sink into this for some time.

When you are ready, come back to your body, but imagine that your body is a doorway. Rather than a place where you live, your body is a doorway where you move from one moment to the next. See if you can imagine and experience your body as a doorway, opening so that you can step through into the next moment, closing behind you, and then opening again in front of you as you move into the next moment. You see, we really don't exist as solid objects fixed in time; we are liminal beings, we are vibrating *spanda*, and we are always on the move, transitioning into the next moment.

BECOMING WHO YOU ARE

> Owning our story and loving ourselves through the process is the bravest thing that we'll ever do.[355]
>
> BRENÉ BROWN

M. Scott Peck writes of the road less traveled (in his book of the same name) as a challenging path of the soul or Self in the process of growing and becoming. Peck points out that the path of growth is difficult. Resistance to accepting difficulties in life can interfere with growth. Essentially, one can end up stuck in the middle of the road one is trying to take, not realizing that there is another road, a road less traveled, that leads uphill. This road may, at first, seem more difficult, but in the long run it could be the more rewarding path. As Robert Frost wrote in the poem "The Road Not Taken," taking the road less traveled "made all the difference."[356]

Before we can become who we are, we sometimes have to get lost and lose who we thought we were supposed to be, or stop trying to be who others want us to be. Rebecca Solnit, in *A Field Guide to Getting Lost*, references a paraphrase of Meno's paradox: "How will you go about finding that thing the nature of which is totally unknown to you?"[357] The answer is getting lost. "The question then," she writes, "is how to get lost. Never to get lost is not to live, not to know how to get lost brings you to destruction, and somewhere in the terra incognita in between lies a life of discovery."[358] Here we are again, back in the liminal space of disorientation. Solnit tells us that *never to get lost is not to live.* Perhaps in burnout and compassion fatigue, when we feel we have lost our souls, this is actually part of living and finding who we are becoming.

> **become** (v.) Old English *becuman* "happen, come about, befall," also "meet with, fall in with; arrive, approach, enter," from Proto-Germanic **bikweman* . . . Meaning "change from one state of existence to another"[359]

We can see from the etymology of the word "become" that becoming involves happenings, enterings, things befalling us, also perhaps meeting someone helpful along the way as we *change from one state of existence to another.*

James Hillman, in his book *The Soul's Code: In Search of Character and Calling*, describes the "acorn theory" of development, which holds that each of us is a unique individual and that our purpose in life is to grow from the potential in the acorn into who we truly can be, or as we might say in this section, *becoming who you are.*

> In a nutshell, then, this book is about calling, about fate, about character, about innate image. Together they make up the "acorn theory," which holds that each person bears a uniqueness that asks to be lived and that is already present before it can be lived.[360]

According to Hillman, "each life is formed by its unique image, an image that is the essence of life and calls it to a destiny . . . this image acts as a personal daimon, an accompanying guide who remembers your calling."[361] When he speaks of a "personal daimon," this Greek term is the same used by Socrates in describing his guiding spirit, what might also be called a guardian angel. Hillman writes that in ancient times, everyone was thought to have an inner guide, a soul, *daimon*, or *genius*. Like Michael Meade (see *The Genius Myth*, discussed in chapter 5), Hillman believes something unique within us is waiting to be born.

Joseph Rael and I have published his teachings for children in our book *Becoming Who You Are*. Joseph was taught at Picuris Pueblo that children are born divine beings, holy beings, and that they are children of the stars. Joseph tells us:

> Becoming who you are *is* about learning, but it's not learning just anything. Becoming who you are is about learning ancient wisdom—knowledge passed down through generations of experience—because the ancient ancestors, just like the Oracle at Delphi, Socrates, and Plato, were always trying to help the next generation of young students to "know thyself," to learn who they are. . . .
>
> Who you are is like a seed, a seed buried and hidden deep within your heart. A seed is a circle, the circle of life, which is another name for the medicine wheel. Everything you do in the world starts with you, goes out into the world, and then comes back again. Seeds grow from the darkness of unknowing into the light of knowing, then blossom, creating more seeds. When you hold

a seed in your hand, it is hard to tell what kind of plant it will grow into, and so it is with you! What kind of human being will you become? *Who are you*?[362]

BECOMING PRACTICE— BECOMING THE STAR OF YOUR OWN LIFE

Take some time to find a comfortable place.

When you are ready, take a few deep breaths.

Sink into the center of yourself. Imagine a bright spark within you that seeks to manifest in the world.

Imagine your birth, how you came into this world.

Imagine yourself as an infant, small and vulnerable, a spark of life in the world.

Next, we will practice remembering and imagining. This remembering will stretch back to years you have already lived, imagining will be imagining time that has not happened yet. Picture yourself at 1-year intervals: 1 year old . . . 2 years old . . . 3 years old. Next by 3-year intervals: 6 years old, 9 years old, 12 years old. Then by 6-year intervals: 18 years old, 24 years old, 30 years old. Next by 9-year intervals: 39 years old, 48 years old, 57 years old. Then by 12-year intervals: 69 years old, 81 years old, 93 years old. Finally, imagine yourself at your oldest.

Imagine a line or thread, stretching through each of these Selves of yours at different times in your life—some kind of colored thread or electrical circuit imagery, connecting all of your Selves across time.

Imagine yourself at your oldest and at your youngest. Imagine you at your oldest reaching back and taking the hand of you at your youngest—this closes the circle of your life, connecting beginning and end. Imagine, as you close this circle, that a tremendous light and heat begins to build up in the center of the circle of your life. Small at first, then expanding out to reach all of your Selves and then expanding beyond all of your Selves, out into the Earth, into space, into the space between things in space. Experience the pulsation of your being emanating light out into the vastness of reality. You are a star. The elements that compose your body came from previous generations of stars, and a star, still, you are.

Take three deep breaths as you rest in the expansiveness of your being. Gradually open your eyes and see if you can bring this awareness of your shining light across time into your day-to-day life. Imagine this inner light illuminating your path of becoming who you are.

10

BECOMING CARING: CARING FOR ALL

Returning—Interbeing—Leading

WITH BECOMING CARING, we are coming full circle, returning after transformation, back to where we started. As in Mezirow's transformative learning, there is a reintegration into life after the disorienting dilemma. We can think of this movement as a spiral, where we return to the "same" place, but in a different orientation, or we can think of it as an ever-widening circle of consciousness, where our circle of responsibility expands from ourselves to include others.

The verb "becoming" initiates us into an ongoing practice of caring. Becoming tells us that we are not there yet—there is still another mountain to climb, another river to cross, a forest to explore—and yet, we are already there, we already have everything we need inside us. We just have to remember that we are not alone, we are all in this together.

In Becoming Caring, we look at three different attributes of Caring for All—*returning* (returning to our calling after strengthening our foundation), *interbeing* (developing a sense of nondual oneness), and finally, *leading* (expanding our caring from self to others).

RETURNING

> To go to the Supreme is a wandering, a wandering afar, and this wandering afar is a returning.[363]
>
> *TAO TE CHING*, VERSE XXV

> *The return and reintegration with society*, which is indispensable to the continuous circulation of spiritual energy into the world, and which, from the standpoint of the community, is the justification of the long retreat, the hero himself may find the most difficult requirement of all.[364]
>
> JOSEPH CAMPBELL

The journey of returning to Self, of recovering your lost soul, of reconnecting "soul and role"[365] (as Parker J. Palmer says), is a completion and a beginning. Journeys of transformation are circular, ending where they began; however, you are transformed in the process. Joseph Campbell's hero's journey model involves a returning of the hero or heroine back into society. However, Campbell found that society often rejects the returning hero or heroine, even though society needs the new perspective and rejuvenation they carry or embody. Part of the challenge of crossing the return threshold is holding fast to one's inner authority to convince society (and oneself) that one has something of value to give.

The hero or heroine is like an empty bowl which becomes full, then out of abundance seeks to give to whomever is thirsty or needing nourishment. After working on self-transformation, one receives insight, peace, and wisdom. Wisdom teaches that one only receives what one is meant to give—like the heart receiving the most oxygen-enriched blood of the body and then giving it away, only to receive back the most depleted blood in the body and then giving it away and completing the cycle over and over again.

Returning to Your Calling

Having a strong sense of meaning and commitment in your work is protective against burnout.[366] Your calling is why you became a healer and teacher. It is the first step in the healer's journey—the call to adventure. Since the journey is a circle, you periodically return to renew your calling, to strengthen your commitment, to renew your oath of *caring for self & others*.

Theologian Matthew Fox created the Order of the Sacred Earth with a very simple oath or vow, and then an explanation of the importance of vows. These explanations of the benefit of taking vows might lead you to review your calling:

> The Vow: "I Promise to Be the Best Lover and Defender of the Earth that I Can Be."
>
> Why do people take vows? When you are distracted, a vow allows you to focus. When you are conflicted, a vow reminds you of the values to which you've committed. When the confusions and problems of life pull you away from your life goal and purpose, a vow clarifies your path. When you are tempted to fall into apathy or despair, a vow challenges you to gather all your energy for a particular and noble purpose. It allows for, indeed calls for, some heavy lifting. A vow deepens your life's path from "job" or "career" to "mission" or "vocation," and supports that vocation in good times and bad . . . a lifeline in these times of global transition.[367]

Did you take an oath or vow as a student or in your professional education, such as the Hippocratic Oath? What might your oath be? How could you put the feeling of your original calling into words? The following are three examples to consider, then try writing your own.

Here is an example of an oath written by the University of Minnesota Medical School class of 2017 during their 2013 orientation:

> In the presence of our families, colleagues, and communities, we take this oath in recognition of the honor and privilege of becoming a physician.
>
> We arrive at the threshold of our chosen profession pledging to preserve our humility, integrity, and all the values which brought us to the practice of medicine. We will engage in honest self-reflection, striving for

> excellence but acknowledging our limitations, and caring for ourselves as we care for others.
>
> We will collaborate with our colleagues, patients, and communities to improve the practice of medicine. We will discover, innovate, learn, and teach as responsible stewards of medical knowledge.
>
> We will seek to heal the whole person rather than merely treat disease, committing to a partnership with our patients that empowers them and demonstrates empathy and respect. We will cure sometimes, treat often, and comfort always.
>
> We will not betray the trust of our patients, who give us the privilege to stand by them in their most vulnerable moments. We will respect diversity in all forms and advocate for the needs of our patients in the context of their lived experiences. We will fight for health equity and social justice on behalf of our patients, our communities, and our world.
>
> Let this Commencement day symbolize the acknowledgment of our own humanity, our dedication to the art and science of medicine, and our responsibility to serve.[368]

How many of these themes resonate with your own calling in health care? Here is another oath to consider, written by physicians Mukta Panda, Kevin O'Brien, and Margaret Lo for the Collaborative for Healing and Renewal in Medicine (CHARM). This oath capitalizes on the guiding principles of the Charter on Physician Well-Being that wellness is a shared responsibility between the individual provider and the system.[369]

Oath to Self-Care and Well-Being

1. We solemnly pledge to embrace and promote
   the well-being of our self, our colleagues, and the
   medical community as part of our responsibility to
   the effective care of our patients, ourselves, and in
   partnership with our healthcare organization.

2. We will seek to develop and adhere to habits that promote and maintain humility, meaning, and wholeness of self in our work and interactions.

3. We will be attuned to the physical, emotional, mental, and spiritual needs of our self and others and share our practices of well-being for the benefits of our patients, our colleagues, and the advancement of healthcare.

4. We will commit to integration and balance in our professional and personal life and seek help when we feel we ourselves or our peers are overburdened, fatigued, or less compassionate.

5. We will champion for a healthcare system that values the well-being of its personnel, uses best evidence for an institutional culture of wellness, and recognizes that in so promoting the patients we care for are ultimately best served.

6. We will find the courage to be vulnerable and confront professional wrongdoings to the best of our ability while at the same time showing compassion and respect for all members of the healthcare team.

7. I make these promises of well-being to myself and to the vocation of medicine with my highest commitment.[370]

Caring for Self & Others Oath

I offer the following oath to bring together the ten dimensions of being fully human, as explored in this book:

> I vow to care for my Self & Others, recognizing that Self includes Others and Others include Self. Therefore, I vow to care for All.
>
> I vow to care for my body and the bodies of others: caring for embodying, animating, and nourishing.

I vow to care for my emotions and the emotions of others: caring for feeling, connecting, and flowing.

I vow to care for my mind and the minds of others: caring for thinking, minding, and evolving.

I vow to care for my heart and the hearts of others: caring for compassioning, loving, and relating.

I vow to care for my creativity and the creativity of others: caring for wording, drawing, and creating.

I vow to care for my intuition and the intuition of others: caring for dreaming, visioning, and receiving.

I vow to care for my spirit and the spirit of others: caring for integrating, unifying, and transforming.

I vow to care for my context and the context of others: caring for harmonizing, sustaining, and communing.

I vow to care for my time and the time of others: caring for growing, transitioning, and becoming who we are.

I vow to care for All, coming full circle and becoming caring: caring for returning, interbeing, and leading caring.

My Calling

As I have worked with my own burnout and soul loss, I have searched back in time for the first inklings of my calling as a healer. I find different beginnings at different times. I imagine this is how it is for many of us complex human beings. I've written elsewhere about a dark night of the soul I went through in college, and how looking at the books on my shelf, such as M. Scott Peck's *The Road Less Traveled* and Jung's *Modern Man in Search of a Soul*, helped me to find the path that led me to medical school and psychiatry.[371] However, something even earlier than college stands out as I have looked back for the beginning of my calling, and I will share it with you now.

When I was young, my mom raised miniature schnauzers, and we often had a litter of puppies in the house and sometimes even two litters. When I was probably around ten or twelve years old, I found myself getting interested in the personalities of the puppies.

From a very young age, some seemed very outgoing and others seemed very shy. I would watch as they would eat when they started on puppy food. The more outgoing puppies wouldn't waste a second getting to the food, sometimes even standing in the food dish as they ate. The puppies that were more shy often got pushed out of the feeding frenzy. As a shy kid myself, I identified with the more reserved puppies.

With one litter, I picked out a particularly shy puppy. I called him Lummie, after the alien creature Lummox in Robert Heinlein's *The Star Beast.* I would make sure Lummie would get first crack at the food and then let the feeding frenzy begin. I would take Lummie out of the pen every day and make sure he got some one-on-one time before playing with the jubilant horde. Over time, Lummie began to be less shy and his quirky personality blossomed.

This was more of an instinctual intervention on my part than a logical scientific experiment. It was done out of love and a sense of justice. Looking back, I consider this one of the formative phases of my calling as a healer—when I developed a practice of caring for those who are marginalized or excluded.

RETURNING PRACTICE—
YOUR OWN CARING FOR SELF & OTHERS OATH

Beautiful Painted Arrow learned from his grandparents that work is worship. In this practice, see if you can notice a sense of seriousness, reverence, or sacredness in your calling. Maybe part of burnout, compassion fatigue, and soul loss is losing touch with your calling. Maybe by practicing embodying your calling, you can reignite your compassion and soul. See if you can find any early memories of your calling to be a healer, educator, or leader.

Find a comfortable posture and place and take a few deep breaths.

Allow your imagination to reach back to the place where your calling started.

Return to your calling, the reason you started on the healer's path.

Beyond thoughts and conscious decisions, allow your whole body to remember what it was like to be alive and buzzing with passion to embark on your healer's journey.

Why did you go into your profession?

What excited you and interested you about it?

Why did you persist through the ups and downs to enter your profession?

Were there any episodes from childhood where you remember becoming aware of a glimmer of your future calling?

Notice the feelings in your body connected with this idealism, passion, and vitality. Notice your emotions around your calling. Notice with your mind, your heart, your expression, your intuition, and your spirit what it feels like to have heard this calling and worked to embody it in your life's work. This feeling of embodying your calling is what it means to be connected to the passions of your soul.

When you burn out, focus on returning to your breath and returning to your calling.

When you experience compassion fatigue, focus on returning to your breath and returning to your calling.

When you have lost your soul, focus on returning to your breath and focus on returning to your calling—your calling is the place where your soul enters you. Maybe it is not your soul that was lost; maybe it was you who forgot your original instructions for bringing your soul into this world.

If you would like, try writing about your calling. If it feels right, you can also draft your own Caring for Self & Others oath to remind you of your calling. Put your inspiration and intention into words. Write it out to make it concrete. Let it sit for a day, a week, and come back to it. See if there is anything else you want to add. This can be your personal oath, your call to vocation. It is precious and has power in it. It is a work of worship. Nurture it, let it grow, and also let it remind you of who you are. You can even make it into a decorated or illustrated certificate to put on the wall.

INTERBEING

In the heat of the Vietnam War, Thich Nhat Hanh established the Buddhist Order of Interbeing. The idea of *interbeing* is that we are all interrelated; there is no self/other, only Self. Thich Nhat Hanh describes the concept: "I am therefore you are. You are, therefore I am. That is the meaning of 'interbeing.' We interare."[372] Our existence depends upon others' existence. In this sense, there is no "self" separated from "other"; all there is, is *interbeing*, because we *interare*. Caring for self is caring for other and caring for other is caring for self. Or, to put it another way, there is no "self" in the absence of "other." Thich Nhat Hanh's concept of interbeing is a nondual perspective of profound interconnection.

The individual practice of meditation leads one from ego to Self to other to All. When the realization of Oneness with the All leads to compassionate action, we have what Thich Nhat Hanh calls *engaged Buddhism*—the practice of meditation in action:

> Once you know what is going on, you're motivated by a desire to do something to relieve the suffering—both in you and around you. And so, we had to find a way to practice mindful breathing and do walking meditation while helping those wounded by bombs—because if you don't maintain a spiritual practice during the time you serve, you will lose yourself and you will burn out.[373]

The work of engaged Buddhism sounds very much like what we are trying to do in health care—we have taken vows and oaths to alleviate suffering, and we seek to engage in the world; however, we may not have the benefit of a spiritual practice integrated within our work. Perhaps what we need in medicine is some kind of spiritual practice as part of our calling and to focus on growing and strengthening what the Buddhists call a *sangha*, a community of practitioners dedicated to seeking the truth, supporting each other, and alleviating suffering.

Charles Eisenstein also writes of interbeing, the "fundamental precept . . . that we are inseparate from the universe, and our being partakes in the being of everyone and everything else."[374] He contrasts the polarized views of activists on the one hand, who say we need to act in the world, and on the other hand, personal growth advocates who say we need to do self-work before other-work. Interbeing, Eisenstein writes, "unites . . . activism and healing."[375] When interbeing breaks down the "rigid self/other distinction, then we recognize that the world mirrors the self; that to work on the self it is necessary to work in the world, and to work effectively in the world, it is necessary to work on the self."[376] In his writing, Eisenstein contrasts two narratives or stories, the *story of separation* and the *story of interbeing*. He sees the story of separation as the root cause of many of the individual and social ills in contemporary society, such as the crises in education, economics, environment, health care, relationships, and addictions.

Charles Foster writes of a similar story of separation. After writing *Being a Beast*, his next book was called *Being a Human*, in which he writes about our cognitive and behavioral separation from the natural world. He sees this as a shrinking of our sense of self and identity where our sense of the "I" becomes the boundaries of our skins, rather than the ecosystems we are part of. Foster studies three different ages in human history, the Upper Paleolithic (35,000–40,000 years ago), the Neolithic (10,000–12,000 years ago), and the Enlightenment (starting around 400 years ago). Foster doesn't just think about things, he tries to experience them in his body. Just as he lived as various animals, such as an otter, a fox, or a badger in *Being a Beast*, he and his son set out to live as close as possible to the ways that an Upper Paleolithic, Neolithic, and Enlightenment person might have lived.

One of the critical elements of being interconnected has to do with soul. In talking about the ancient city of Jericho, a place that was an early adopter of the Neolithic shift from a hunter-gatherer society to an agrarian society, Foster muses:

> Perhaps it was here that animals first started to be seen as things rather than fellow-travellers; here that the process of de-souling the non-human world began. Perhaps the idea of ownership was conceived here: of title and hence entitlement. Perhaps here, having partially de-souled the non-human world, the process of de-souling other humans started.[377]

While spiritual traditions support the evolution of consciousness *forward* into more inclusive realms of interbeing and Oneness, Foster points out that human beings may have already been living in a greater state of interconnectedness in the past. Our movement "forward" in interbeing may be, in some way, a return to our origins.

Could the scientific "advance" of banishing the soul from our identities as educated professionals in the twenty-first century actually contribute to burnout and soul loss? Could the *story of separation* make the costs of caring worse? Could the *story of separation* contribute to burnout, compassion fatigue, and soul loss? Without a supportive and nurturing network of interbeing, we are each alone in a complex and overwhelming world, but if we *interare*, we are all in this together, we have each other's backs, and we have each other's support.

Interbeing is also related to King's Beloved Community. "Interconnectedness—*interbeing* in Nhat Hanh's usage—is central to the understanding of the Beloved Community," writes Marc Andrus in his book *Brothers in the Beloved Community: The Friendship of Thich Nhat Hanh and Martin Luther King Jr.*[378] After Dr. King's assassination, Thich Nhat Hanh vowed to continue the work of the Beloved Community. Additionally, he added a focus on gender equality, expanded the Beloved Community to all life, not just human life, and he blended in the practice of mindfulness for promoting universal peace and justice.

Rediscovering the Joy of Caring: Compassion as an Antidote to Burnout

Interbeing and the Beloved Community just might be the medicine that we need as the antidote to the costs of caring. Theologian Henri Nouwen wrote, "The joy that compassion brings is one of the best-kept secrets of humanity. It is a secret known only to a few people, a secret that has to be rediscovered again and again."[379] How can we work to rediscover the secret of compassion in health care? What does *interbeing* mean, practically, in the work of health care?

Trzeciak and Mazzarelli's review of the literature on compassion suggests "compassion as an antidote to burnout," meaning that the "real antidote to burnout is *leaning in* rather than pulling back" from clinical care.

> However, the preponderance of the data in the scientific literature . . . shows that human connection can transform the experience for the giver of compassion, trigger positive emotion, and build resilience.[380]

Trzeciak and Mazzarelli define compassion as "the emotional response to another's pain or suffering, involving an authentic desire to help."[381] Compassion is as much an action as it is a feeling. If we solely focus on our own feelings of burnout or compassion fatigue, we are still viewing ourselves as isolated and viewing compassion as a limited commodity.

This can seem counter-intuitive; if we are burnt out, our compassion is empty, so we need to pull back, to take care of ourselves, don't we? Maybe short-term, but then we need to get back in the game, we need to get back on the horse. Trzeciak and Mazzarelli warn that the narrative of individual self-care as "escapism" can be isolating and doesn't solve the issues in the workplace that led to burnout in the first place.

> The answer to workplace burnout could not be to run away from the workplace. How was that a sustainable strategy for me, as the head of my department? Something had to change fundamentally at the point of care to reverse my, and anyone's, disconnection, emotional exhaustion, and hopelessness.[382]

The authors point out that there is a paradox that "serving others benefits *you*." This is the focus of their second book, *Wonder Drug: 7 Scientifically Proven Ways that Serving Others Is the Best Medicine for Yourself*. Trzeciak and Mazzarelli are scientists—they are not making a philosophical or humanistic argument. They reviewed the science on caring and compassion and found that it tells us that caring for others is caring for ourselves. The science supports interbeing.

Jean Watson has made a life's work of studying caring and developing Unitary Caring Science. As I mentioned in chapter 9, Watson's description of caring is transpersonal, extending beyond the individual and linking us into an interconnected web. Caring shifts us from separate individual into interbeing.

> We cannot know caring unless we have learned it from within, for our self, with our self, and with others—within a relational world view. Human caring begins with a love of self and other, of humanity and all living things—opening and welcoming the immanent and the transcendent, the subtle, radiant, shadow-and-light, vicissitudes of experiences of embodied living, dying, growing, changing, evolving; honoring with reverence the mystery, miracles, paradoxes, unknowns, the impermanence of changes while still actively, joyfully participating in all of it: the pain, the joy, and everything.[383]

INTERBEING PRACTICE—NONDUAL CARING

I invite you to find a comfortable meditation position; you can even lie down for this one.

Notice the sensations in your body as you slowly scan from head to toes: face, head, neck, shoulders, back, arms, fingers, torso, abdomen, pelvis, legs, feet, and toes. Bring your attention to your fingertips and toe tips and the whole periphery of your body and the insides of your body. Notice your whole body, internally and externally. Notice your body and that you are more than your physical body.

Notice any emotions and feelings present and observe where they are located within your body. Give yourself over to your emotions, letting them crest and trough like ocean waves, coming and going, bringing information about the inner and outer worlds. Notice your emotions and that there is more to you than just your emotions.

Focus on your mind, your thoughts. Notice what happens with your body and emotions as different thoughts pass through you, like leaves floating on a meandering stream. Notice your mind and that there is more to you than just your thoughts. There is the part of you thinking thoughts and the part of you minding and observing yourself thinking.

Bring your attention to your heart, allowing your heart to gently open. You might feel pain, suffering, or sadness when working with your heart at times—that is okay. You may feel joy and happiness at times when working with your heart—that is okay, too. Imagine your heart pumping, circulating your lifeblood. Feel the strength of your heart within you, constantly working for change.

Shift your focus to your throat. Feel the potential of everything buried within you, waiting to be brought into the world. Connect to the essence of who you are and what you must express in this world.

Bring your attention to your forehead, to your place of intuition, of inner knowing and connection. Allow intuition to arise within you.

Shift your focus to the top of your head and feel your spiritual connection to the larger universe.

In your journey from toes to head, you move from the personal to the universal; like a tree growing toward the sun, your uppermost branches are reaching for (en)light(enment).

Allow your attention to shift to your context—the physical, interpersonal, and natural world around you. Notice your interconnection with all things.

Bring your attention to the river of time within which you are immersed. Feel the flow of time, carrying you along on your journey. Moment to moment, day to day, week to week, month to month, year to year—you are a being in movement, flowing, swimming, journeying through time.

If you would like, take a pause, allow yourself to melt like butter, shifting from your sense of separation and becoming one with the dough of life. Instead of me and mine, feel the presence of we and our. Allow the presence of life, the world, everything as it is, a state of interbeing with all life. Feel the Beloved Community of humanity, the Beloved Community of all the children of Mother Earth.

Rest easily.

Take a few deep breaths.

Sense the movement of life within you and all you share this Earth with. Feel into that which you share with all beings.

Sense how your suffering affects those around you and how others' suffering affects you as well.

Sense how your joy affects those around you and how others' joy affects you as well. Feel into your interbeing because you and all around you interare.

When you are ready, invite your heart and the hearts of all the world into interbeing. Take a few deep breaths. Slowly open your eyes and feel the gratitude and support that comes from interbeing.

LEADING CARING

> Any idiot can face a crisis; it's this day-to-day living that wears you out.[384]
>
> ANONYMOUS

How can we lead caring when caring is difficult to count and measure? How can we take the time to care when there are so many other demands and metrics to meet? Schwartz and colleagues tell us that leaders are asking the wrong questions:

> "How can we get more out of our people?" leaders regularly ask us. We suggest they pose a different question: "How can I more intentionally invest in meeting the multidimensional needs of my employees so they're freed, fueled, and inspired to bring the best of themselves to work every day?"
>
> To build competitive advantage, organizations must help employees cultivate qualities that have never before been critical—among them authenticity, empathy, self-awareness, constant creativity, and internal sense of purpose, and, perhaps above all, resilience in the face of relentless change.[385]

While Schwartz works in the larger business world, a similar argument is made by Spiegelman and Berrett in their book *Patients Come Second: Leading Change by Changing the Way You Lead.* We cannot expect health care workers to give what they don't have. As I said in the beginning of the book, you have to put on your own oxygen mask before you can help others.

All of us are leaders in different ways. In *Re-humanizing Medicine,* I outlined three levels of leadership: *internal, professional,* and *organizational.* When we think of leadership, we usually think of someone who is in charge of others, managing and directing groups. Yet, as we have seen in looking at the dimensions of Self, we are each composed of a variety of dimensions that can have conflicting or synergistic relationships. In this way, we are all the leaders of a very complex organization—a human being. Bringing our human elements into harmony is *internal leadership. Professional leadership* is what occurs in small groups or in one-on-one relationships, in the clinics, the classrooms, and businesses. You may not be in a formal leadership role, but when we function as professionals, there is an inherent moral and ethical leadership we are embodying in serving others. *Organizational leadership* is what we usually think of as traditional leadership—directors, team leads, CEOs—providing guidance and direction of large groups.

Holistic leadership brings together these three levels of leadership: internal, professional, and organizational. Holistic leadership integrates internal dimensions and external dimensions, creating a framework that supports "human growth and healing within complex systems."[386] Just as we often say in medicine that the ideal system builds itself around the needs of the patient, so too the ideal institution builds itself around the human needs of the individuals working within that institution. Thus, holistic leadership aims to transform the culture of medicine through awareness of human needs.

The Limits of Self-Care

The challenge comes in creating a culture of caring that supports human being. In Medscape's 2023 survey of physician burnout, the top six reasons given for burnout did not directly involve working with patients. Physicians listed bureaucracy, lack of respect from administration and colleagues, too many hours at work, lack of autonomy, insufficient compensation, and the stress of electronic medical health records before they even mentioned any issues with patients.[387] Maybe burnout is not caused by too much caring and compassion going out, but rather too much institutional interference with our ability to connect to ourselves—and through ourselves connect to others. The modern practice of medicine can feel more like trying to run a call center with phone calls, emails, secure messages, multiple team message threads, electronic record alerts, and computer charting requirements in which it is easy to lose our souls—and when we have lost our souls, there is no way we can connect to the soul of another. It is not that we are doing too much caring at work, but rather we are not doing enough caring at work—those logistics feel like everything but personal caring. Is there a way to better care for health care workers so that they can better care for others?

When practiced in isolation from others, our self-care practices seek to replenish us without restoring a sense of interconnectedness or nonduality. Caring for ourselves can become yet another protocol we are trying to implement and manage by pulling away from the world into our isolated egos. When we try to build up the ego-system of our bodies, emotions, and minds, we view caring as a zero-sum game, as a limited commodity. In contrast, ecosystems of our souls include all other beings and the Earth herself. If you are working in a system that is not caring for you, and there is no room to work on transforming the system, leaving may be the best medicine for you. This is what many workers in health care, teaching, and many other fields are deciding, and this has been called "the great resignation."

Personally, I have worked in fourteen different organizations over the course of my career. Sometimes I left because of a move to a different part of the country or a different part of the world, or for a job opportunity. There have been a few times, however, that I left because a job was beginning to feel soul crushing or because I was increasingly feeling a values conflict between the organization and my professional identity. I turned down a medical directorship that did not seem to have any authority or responsibility beyond being a figurehead for the org chart. I turned down an opportunity to be the head of a department that involved "cutting out the dead wood" and "cherry-picking insurance contracts." That really meant getting rid of my friends and colleagues and dropping Medicaid patients. I ended up leaving an organization that was physician-owned for years after the clinic was sold to an outside medical management firm that wanted us to shift from a Relative Value Unit (RVU) model of income parity for physicians to what they literally called an "eat what you kill" model. I have written about that decision in *Re-humanizing Medicine* where I decided that the moral cost of staying in the organization outweighed my fear of the unknown and the onerous two-year, 30-mile non-compete clause I had to work around.[388]

There are times where there is a leadership change or a change in your life situation where it makes sense to think about leaving for another job. However, many of the institutional determinants of clinician wellness are found within many practices. You could end up jumping out of the frying pan and into the fire. Every job has strengths and weaknesses. For instance, at one point, I stopped being an employee and started my own holistic psychiatry private practice. I had a great deal of flexibility, but I had so much more responsibility for scheduling and billing, and if I took a vacation, I did not get paid. Working at the VA now, I have tremendous support as a federal employee with sick leave, vacation leave, and benefits—but sometimes I feel like I am paying with my soul, as the bureaucracy can sometimes make it feel like a layer of my soul is sand-papered off every year.

In my private practice I over-extended myself several times. I couldn't blame someone else for my burnout and feeling overworked (although I would often say that my boss made me work evenings and weekends). Even doing holistic psychiatry, focusing on self-care and wellness for clients, I was overworking—I came to call it the "holistic death march." I was doing too much, even though it was a good thing that I was doing, and I was not enjoying it—burnout!

Working with Whole Health at the VA, I have similarly worked myself into Whole Health Burnout several times. I have learned that even when working with a wellness perspective, it is easy to burn out from too much wellness work! I have felt ashamed and stupid when I get myself into those situations of burning out from being over-extended, but health care systems seem to run on over-extension, even when you are your own boss. Maybe if I had been doing more self-care and taking better care of myself and told people "no" instead of "yes," I would not have burned out?

Barton and colleagues warn that the "emphasis on self-care may undermine, rather than support, employee wellness," because health, particularly at work, is not an individual issue—rather "our psychological health is grounded in attachment to and acceptance by others." The authors further state, "Rather than focusing on *self-care*, we need to be better at *taking care of each other* . . . framing employee distress as a collective rather than individual problem."[389] Their argument is similar to work coming out of the health care field that we will review next, asserting that burnout is not an individual problem, but an institutional issue.

Taking care of each other is exactly what we are trying to do in *Caring for Self & Others*, recognizing that we *interare*—we are all in this together. Interbeing reminds us that we are only as healthy as those around us and that the suffering of one is the suffering of all. Likewise, true caring means that the care of one is also the care of all. Suffering is collective, not individual. The solution in the workplace, according to Barton and colleagues, is to create a "relational pause," a space for emotions and caring, leading to "acknowledging our collective ownership of suffering."[390]

Beyond Resilience to System Transformation

While resilience and self-care are part of the puzzle for recovering from burnout and soul loss, to only focus on these individual responsibilities runs the risk of blaming the victim. Are high rates of burnout actually due to the way our systems are designed? Swensen and Shanafelt think so, writing that the "current health care delivery system is perfectly designed to create high rates of professional burnout in physicians, nurses, advanced practice providers, and other health care professionals."[391] The problem, then, is not a lack of resilience within staff, but an institutional structure that does not support human flourishing. To address burnout and compassion fatigue, we have to go beyond individual resilience.[392]

> **resilience** (n.) "act of rebounding". . . from Latin *resiliens*, present participle of *resilire* "to rebound, recoil," from *re-* "back". . . + *salire* "to jump, leap"[393]

While the ability to bounce back is important, we also need to transform, which means to grow beyond our previous limits. Transformation means we are not trying to be who we were, rather we are growing into the potential of who we can become. Many are questioning whether resilience is really the answer to the burnout pandemic, particularly within the field of posttraumatic growth. As Edith Shiro writes in *The Unexpected Gift of Trauma: The Path to Posttraumatic Growth*, "resilience doesn't help us *grow* from adversity, it helps us *cope* with it, and further, "sometimes resilience actually hinders the possibility of achieving" posttraumatic growth.[394]

Richard Tedeschi and Lawrence Calhoun have been studying posttraumatic growth for years and they point out that "continuing personal distress and growth often coexist."[395] In this sense, the goal is not to be free of suffering, but to grow from it. This distinguishes a transformative growth paradigm from the prevention and recovery focus on work-readiness of the resilience paradigm. Rather than bouncing back to our previous level of adaptation, transformation helps us grow beyond it. Just as Chenrezig was not put back together with two arms and two eyes, we want to grow in the ability to see and touch suffering. Tedeschi and Calhoun describe posttraumatic growth as an experience where development "has surpassed what was present before the struggle with crises occurred," and that this is not "simply a return to baseline—it is an experience of improvement that for some persons is deeply profound." Posttraumatic growth "has a quality of transformation . . . unlike . . . resilience."[396]

Resilience and subjective well-being can be part of the approach to burnout, compassion fatigue, and soul loss, but only take us so far—they can restore previous functioning, but do not help us grow as healers or as human beings. Posttraumatic growth and post-burnout growth are transformation paradigms that take us beyond resilience, however we still need to look beyond the individual to the health care ecosystems we work in and the institutional variables that contribute to burnout, maintain it, and limit our focus to being the same productive work unit we were yesterday instead of supporting a transformational growth mindset.

It is worth re-examining the costs of caring again, this time looking at the systemic and organizational issues, as we have been covering the personal and individual levels. We can look at the costs of caring from a different perspective after taking the journey of caring for self & others. Each cost incurs an aspect of suffering but can also be seen as having a joyful counterpart: from burnout to post-burnout growth, from trauma to posttraumatic growth, from dehumanization to re-humanization, from demoralization to remoralization, from soul loss to soul recovery, and from suicide to finding meaning and purpose which leads to joy and flourishing. It is not easy work to dig ourselves out of the abyss of the *costs of caring* and to return, transformed, back into the health care world, armed with our rejuvenated *joys of caring*.

Working with people is stressful and exposes us to direct and vicarious trauma. We can't eliminate exposure to suffering from our work. But we can build in ways to grow in our capacity for caring—this doesn't mean never suffering, but developing a greater capacity to work with suffering. In addition to individual approaches, we also need to go beyond resilience to create organizations that measure employee idealism and well-being as well as measuring productivity. As the late Alessandra Pigni, a former Doctors Without Borders psychologist, stated:

> But is self-care enough to prevent burnout? Yes and no. There is self-care as in "a day at the spa," recreational self-care, and there is self-care as "care of the self," a deeper kind of attention to ourselves, the sort that asks questions like, "What am I doing in this group/organization/community? Do I still belong here?" We call this transformational self-care.[397]

Transformational "care of the self" challenges us to look not just at ourselves as individuals, but how we fit in the larger institution. If an institution is not supporting our humanity and for whatever reason we are not able or in a position to transform the institution, that may mean we care for ourselves by changing jobs. If transformation is possible, then we roll up our sleeves and contribute to the challenging work of transforming systems and institutions.

From the beginning, Maslach's work on burnout focused on the relationship between the individual and the institution. We are seeing a consensus that burnout is a systems issue—self-care has a role to play, but the real drivers of burnout are institutional variables, as Mayo Clinic's Swensen and Shanafelt conclude:

> It should be emphasized that burnout is mainly caused by systems, leaders, and characteristics of the work environment, not by a deficiency in personal well-being or resilience. When leaders begin the quest to address burnout in their organizations, they often make the mistake of starting individual-focused programs that imply the cause of burnout is due to a lack of resilience on the part of the health care professional . . . this approach leaves staff with an unintended message: They are at fault for their burnout because they have not taken care of themselves.[398]

Burnout is thus a leadership and institutional issue and to put the responsibility solely on the individual professional is what Swensen and Shanafelt call the "strong worker" fallacy. Further, they write, "burnout is primarily the result of health care systems that take emotionally healthy, altruistic people and methodically squeeze the vitality and passion out of them."[399] They describe twelve strategies in their book, building on Shanafelt and Noseworthy's earlier paper which outlined nine strategies for leadership to address burnout at an institutional level.[400]

Thus, we can start with individual self-care to address burnout and the costs of caring, but that is just the start because transformation is required at all levels of the system. Leaders are individuals, too, and when they learn and engage in regular self-care, and lead by example, they can have a powerful impact on the culture. Leaders who know the value of self & other care are more likely to lead in a caring way. Leadership is an act of moral courage. Just to be a professional is to be a moral agent in the world. One of the tasks of leadership is to create a work environment that is designed to create the joys of caring rather than the costs of caring.

Moral Injury & the Institutional Determinants of Clinician Health

> Burnout is the place where ethics and psychology collide. Where we feel moral distress over what we know is the right thing to do, but we are unable to do it because of organizational policies, rules, and office politics.[401]
>
> ALESSANDRA PIGNI

The term "burnout" can disempower the individual, implying they are responsible for the dehumanizing effects of work environments. When our pain is turned into a "syndrome" that is then "managed," our personal narrative and experience is co-opted and turned into some kind of medico-business speak. When lingo replaces human caring, it becomes difficult to remain fully human in a work environment. This is what Samuel Shem's character, Roy, objects to when reductionistic terminology is used to describe his experience. He calls this a "high-ass theory of my pain."[402] Sometimes it is more important to sit with suffering, rather than to try to diagnose, name, or explain it away.

Simon Talbot and Wendy Dean introduce another perspective for looking at the adverse impact of the institutional environment on clinicians—moral injury rather than burnout for understanding physician suffering.

> But the concept of burnout resonates poorly with physicians: it suggests a failure of resourcefulness and resilience, traits that most physicians have finely honed during decades of intense training and demanding work. Even at the Mayo Clinic, which has been tracking, investigating, and addressing burnout for more than a decade, one-third of physicians report its symptoms.

> We believe that burnout is itself a symptom of something larger: our broken health care system. The increasingly complex web of providers' highly conflicted allegiances—to patients, to self, and to employers—and its attendant moral injury may be driving the health care ecosystem to a tipping point and causing the collapse of resilience.[403]

Many physicians embraced their redefinition of health worker suffering from burnout to moral injury, including Zubin Damania (ZDogg MD) and William E. Flanary (Dr. Glaucomflecken). ZDogg picked up Talbot and Dean's story and published a scathing video blog entitled "It's Not Burnout, It's Moral Injury" in 2019.[404] Flanary, as Dr. Glaucomflecken, has posted numerous short videos lampooning the way that institutional leaders fumble with worker burnout.[405] Even US Surgeon General Vivek Murthy appeared as a guest to address burnout with Dr. Glaucomflecken.[406]

The idea of moral injury comes from combat veterans who experienced moral dilemmas or felt morally betrayed by their command. Sonya Norman and Shira Maguen summarize the concept of moral injury:

- When someone does something that goes against their beliefs (an act of commission)
- When they fail to do something in line with their beliefs (an act of omission)
- Individuals may also experience betrayal from leadership, others in positions of power, or peers
- Moral injury is the distressing psychological, behavioral, social, and sometimes spiritual aftermath of exposure to such events
- Moral injury can occur in response to acting or witnessing behaviors that go against an individual's values and moral beliefs[407]

The strain of trying to do the right thing and apply the best level of clinical care within an institution that sets up competing and conflicting demands with professional responsibility can lead to the moral injury spectrum. When computers get more of our time than patients, something is amiss within the health care system. During the pandemic especially, health care professionals have often been in situations where they are under-resourced, where political propaganda and anti-science rhetoric is interfering with public health recommendations, and they are forced to make resource allocation decisions that potentially result in the death of patients. Recognizing this occupational strain, the National Center for PTSD has developed a resource page for moral injury in health care workers.[408]

A year after their ground-breaking article, Dean and Talbot reviewed the response to the concept of moral injury in health care. They called for changing the institution of medicine and honoring and supporting the doctor-patient relationship:

> The long-term solutions to moral injury demand changes in the business framework of health care. The solutions reside not in promoting mindfulness or resilience among individual physicians, but in creating a health care environment that finally acknowledges the value of the time clinicians and patients spend together developing the trust, understanding, and compassion that accompany a true relationship.[409]

The shift from looking at health care worker suffering as an individual deficit (burnout) to an occupational hazard (moral injury) has resonated with many in health care. Rather than looking at only individual self-care, we need institutions that care for staff; rather than only individual resilience, we need organizational transformation into human-centric systems. Whether we call it burnout or moral injury, we need to look at the institutional determinants of physician, clinician, and health care worker health. Our work environments play a role in our health and well-being.

Moral Resilience & Re-moralizing Health Care

Cynda Hylton Rushton has dedicated her career to studying moral injury and how to build moral resilience in systems. She has mapped out a pathway of gradual steps that lead to moral injury: moral adversity, imperiled integrity, moral stress, moral suffering, moral distress, moral outrage, moral injury, and moral decline. She has also plotted a pathway of repair and intervention points: moral repair, integrity, and moral resilience.[410] Rushton reconceptualizes suffering as something that is inherent to life and the work of working with others.

> [Our suffering] must be skillfully worked so that we can transform it to fuel a future of integrity and compassion rather than allow it to disable our basic human goodness and moral community. Rather than seeing our suffering as a weakness, we can view it as a raw material that is needed to build strength and resilience that we can leverage to sustain our integrity, caring practices, clinical expertise, and well-being so that our patients and their loved ones receive quality, safe, and compassionate care.[411]

Rushton sees caring for others as a "moral concern for them as persons and for their well-being and a commitment to take action on their behalf to reduce or relieve their suffering."[412] This view strengthens the role of professionals as "moral agents."

Systems and institutions are fundamentally amoral (incapable of taking moral action) because morality is a human capacity, not a capacity of an institutional flow chart. In this way, professionals hold the moral responsibility within systems. One of the roles of the professional is to be the moral compass for the institution. As Rushton states, "Clinicians have the expertise and moral obligation to advocate for change."[413]

> The goal is to support clinicians to transform their moral suffering with the capacities of moral resilience so that they can serve the people they are dedicated to with greater compassion, wisdom, and ease. This cannot occur

> without fundamental shifts within our healthcare organizations and society.[414]

Rushton recommends system transformation in a synergistic dynamic with personal transformation. Personal transformation drives system transformation and system transformation drives more personal transformation. Transformational leadership is a buzz word, but true transformation means that leaders are attending to their own full humanity (body, emotions, mind, heart, creativity, intuition, spirit, context and environment, and time) as well as the humanity of the people they lead. To create a new narrative to develop moral resilience in ourselves and in our institutions, Rushton suggests:

- Begin by expanding heart space and inner potential
- Adopt personal reflection and insight as the pathway to concise, clear expression
- Connect your initiatives with a shift to a larger purpose
- Help others see their own possibilities for co-creation
- Choose words with intentions and care
- Open and foster space for synergy to emerge
- Focus on and magnify your connection to what you stand for in life
- Enable risk in connecting to your moral compass [415]

We can look at moral injury as overlapping with burnout, compassion fatigue, and soul loss. When someone feels a sense of moral injury in the workplace, they feel alienated, marginalized, silenced, and they can feel they are betraying their values, morals, and professionalism. In working with burnout or soul loss as a personal issue, we need to figure out how to reignite our pilot light, or how to reconnect with our soul's animating abilities. In working with moral injury, we need to focus on *remoralization* to counter demoralization. We can take some individual steps to support remoralization, but it is fundamentally a relational and institutional issue.

Remoralization is a key component of Leading Caring. It is related to restoring hope, validating pain, and being grateful for not only someone's work, but for people's humanity. Caring for another's humanity involves cultivating one's own humanity and then accessing another's humanity through one's own humanity. Remoralization means caring for body, emotions, mind, heart, creativity, intuition, spirit, context, and time. For leaders, you have to be fully human before you can support the full humanity of another.

Medical & Professional Activism

If we go *beyond resilience* as holistic leaders, then we need to transform the system. This is what I mean by activism—not simply working within the systems we find ourselves in, but seeing that our identity as professionals involves a feedback loop of changing the systems within which we work.

This entails a shift or expansion in our professional identities, growing beyond a focus of responsibility within the clinic, the classroom, or the office, to looking at the larger systems we work within—institutional, organizational, political, and global.

Parker J. Palmer has written extensively about "educating the new professional," which he describes as "a person who not only is competent in his or her discipline but also has the skill and the will to resist and help transform the institutional pathologies that threaten the profession's highest standards."[416] The new professional has a moral and ethical responsibility within the institution and cannot hide behind "I just work here," or "it's not my responsibility." Palmer writes that "the education of the new professional would not teach emotional distancing as a strategy for survival. Instead it would teach students to stay close to emotions that might become sources of energy to challenge and change institutions."[417]

A similar concept is that of the "witnessing professional," developed by psychiatrist Robert Jay Lifton. I did an interview with Lifton in 2021, in which he discussed his studies on how totalitarian regimes can create a "malignant normality" where the abnormal becomes gradually accepted as normal. Professionals, such as the Nazi doctors he studied, are not immune to being swept up in social and political movements where they betray their ideals and professional duties to harm others. Lifton suggested that we re-invigorate professionalism to become "witnessing professionals," who recognize a moral obligation to uphold ideals and values. The concept of witnessing comes out of trauma and human rights work. "There is an increasing recognition on the part of many professionals that what they are doing and thinking is not enough and there is a hunger among professionals . . . for . . . including an ethical or moral perspective in their professional work,"[418] Lifton told me.

When we have this sense that we need to do more for the health of our patients and the population, what exactly can we do? John Launer wrote that "Medicine and politics are inseparable"[419] and he argues that activism is an important part of our identity as physicians.

I have been writing and speaking about the topic of medical activism over the last few years.[420] Writing as a physician, I consider medical activism as a subset of *professional activism*. For me, issues around political human rights, the fascist trend in national and world politics, gun violence, environmental issues, and the compassion and burnout crisis in health care have all ignited my passion to make the world a better place. Although physicians and health care workers are sometimes encouraged to "stay in their lane" and function in a narrowly defined role as technicians in the health care assembly line, I believe that we have a greater calling to be *new professionals* and *witnessing professionals*. For me, medical activism comes out of a broad definition of professional identity and also the spiritual insight of interbeing.

I do not in any way mean to overstate my role as a medical activist—I can always do more, we all can always do more. Just as with the story of Chenrezig, there is always more suffering to alleviate, at an individual, societal, global, and environmental level. I hope that this book, in some small way, can contribute to a sense of medical activism, the compassion revolution, and the counter-curriculum of self & other care. Medical activism is when we go beyond the four clinic walls and venture out into the larger world to promote the health of everyone, not only the person in front of us in the consulting room.

Domains of Medical Activism

- Public health
- Social/Moral determinants of health

- Gun violence as a public health issue
- Racism and health, abolition medicine
- Decolonizing medicine
- Religious tolerance
- Human rights medicine and international trauma work
- LGBTQIA+ rights
- Women's rights and reproductive rights
- Immigration health
- Preventing nuclear war
- Peace work, recovery from war and violence
- Climate medicine, animal and plant diversity, environmental health
- Environmental toxins and population health
- Medical student education: preserving idealism and preventing cynicism
- Burnout and moral injury in physicians and health care workers
- Authoritarianism, fascism, and public health

Mona Hanna-Attisha's book *What the Eyes Don't See* describes her advocacy work on the water crisis in Flint, Michigan, and is an example of medical activism. I would also include Dr. Bandy Lee's work as a psychiatrist exercising a duty to warn society of the dangerousness of Donald Trump. Dr. Lee formed the World Coalition of Mental Health and authored and edited two books, *The Dangerous Case of Donald Trump: 37 Psychiatrists and Mental Health Experts Assess a President* and *Profile of a Nation: Trump's Mind, America's Soul*. The thing about medical activism is that you are often pushing against power that has a vested interest to keep things as they are, despite the fact that their actions may be hurting the health of the population. Bandy Lee lost her job at Yale over a narrow interpretation of the Goldwater Rule that psychiatrists are not supposed to speculate about the mental health of public figures. Dr. Lee's argument was that, as a forensic psychiatrist, she has a duty to warn about dangerousness to the public. She argued that the role of professionals as moral agents superseded a limited, technical view of our roles and responsibilities:

> As a psychiatrist, I believe there is no greater oppression than the hijacking of the mind, and critical information at a critical time is necessary to empower the public to be able to protect itself and to act while it is still possible. It is always easier to prevent than to try to limit losses after a problem has become barely containable . . . professionals are supposed to act according to principles of their field as their own moral agents, not as technicians who follow fiats. The latter, a form of ceding one's autonomy, is a formula for becoming an instrument of authoritarianism if not careful. I maintain the humanitarian goals of medicine and our practice of giving precedence to human lives and safety above all else override any etiquette I owe a public figure. This is why the Declaration of Geneva was established, and what the Nuremberg trials were for; we were never supposed to privilege a powerful political figure . . . above the foremost principles of medical ethics to which we have pledged. The mind is considered tyranny's battleground because thought reform occurs through "milieu control," or the control of information in the environment. Most of this has been done through the spread of false information, but we have the chance to change it through a better understanding of truth.[421]

I have a lot of respect for Dr. Lee and I share her definition of professionalism. As the Trump administration devolved over four years, I felt increasingly compelled to write a series of essays called "Words Create Worlds"[422] and publish them on my blog. I immersed myself in readings on fascism, such as Jason Stanley's *How Fascism Works*, Anne Applebaum's *Twilight of Democracy*, Timothy Snyder's *The Road to Unfreedom*, and Madeleine Albright's *Fascism: A Warning*. I couldn't understand why other people didn't see the public health risks of the words of a president that were dehumanizing others and seemed to provoke violence. I took the title of the series of essays from a quote by Susannah Heschel, speaking of her father Rabbi Abraham Joshua Heschel (whom I quoted previously in chapter 5):

> Words, he often wrote, are themselves sacred, God's tool for creating the universe, and our tools for bringing holiness—or evil—into the world. He used to remind us that the Holocaust did not begin with the building of crematoria, and Hitler did not come to power with tanks and guns; it all began with uttering evil words, with defamation, with language and propaganda. Words create worlds he used to tell me when I was a child. They must be used very carefully. Some words, once having been uttered, gain eternity and can never be withdrawn. The Book of Proverbs reminds us, he wrote, that death and life are in the power of the tongue.[423]

I am not interested in politics so much as I am interested in human rights and in overcoming the obstacles to supporting the humanity of everyone. When I spoke with Robert Jay Lifton, I was interested in his thoughts on whether the identity of a witnessing professional is innate in medical students and how much it can be taught. The roots of my own interest in human rights go back to when I was a teenager and interested in punk rock bands with a social conscience advocating for peace, human rights, the environment, and animal rights. Earlier, in my childhood, I grew up with parents who cared for plants and animals and would take in injured animals.

In my medical and psychiatric education at University of Illinois, I worked with Dr. Deb Klamen, and we published a number of papers that could be considered to have a medical activist focus. We published on posttraumatic stress symptoms in medical trainees related to their internship year, and medical student attitudes toward abortion, homosexuality, and AIDS. My work with Stevan Weine during my psychiatry residency was deeply formative. I still hear Steve's voice telling me to be careful with my words, to not fall into the use of technical jargon, and his exhortations to not be satisfied with over-used technical terms that distance us from human suffering. Steve's work was in human rights psychiatry working with Bosnian refugees and he put together a Trauma Studies lecture series that brought together authors, artists, biographers, psychiatrists, and human rights workers.

When I was doing my medical education in Chicago, Quentin Young's work on health care reform was always in the background; I saw him speak and heard him on WBEZ, Chicago Public Radio. Young's biography, *Everybody In, Nobody Out: Memoirs of a Rebel Without a Pause*, documents his work at Cook County Hospital, his support of a single-payer health care plan, and his civil rights work, including marching with Dr. King. Young's words inspired me to join Physicians for a National Health Program and take interest in the politics and economics of health care. I took a two-week elective in health care reform during the fourth year of medical school during the time the Clinton administration was working on the issue. I lived and worked in New Zealand for over three years and had a chance to learn what it was like to work in a national health system.

Another inspirational figure from my education was psychiatrist Carl Bell, who was on faculty at University of Illinois Chicago, where I was doing my residency. He was another tireless activist for underserved populations in Chicago and advocated out-of-the-box thinking. He argued that racism is a health issue that is in psychiatry's lane. Dr. Bell was a social and community psychiatrist who believed that the work of a psychiatrist did not end at the clinic walls but extended out into the community. Here is his critique of psychiatry and the benefit of having a broader, humanistic perspective and responsibility:

> I've recently realized that a major problem with psychiatry is that it's too focused on what we were trained to do. It sometimes feels like psychiatry is stuck in a box that only recognizes diagnosis and treatment. Unfortunately, being in this box precludes psychiatrists from involving themselves with prevention and from focusing on strengths and characteristics of resilience and resistance. These are just as much a part of the human condition as is the psychopathology we were trained to identify and treat. Fortunately, some of us are blessed enough to be on the fringe, which allows us to occasionally leave the box and get a different perspective. This brings new paradigms and models that benefit the human condition.[424]

This idea that our training can blind us to important human dimensions of health and suffering is one I have struggled with much of my career. I also feel like I have often gravitated to the fringe, sometimes working from the outside in and other times working from the inside out. I've come to think of myself as an insider-outsider (or an outsider-insider). The idea of having a calling to leave the comfortable confines of the everyday known world and to venture into the unknown is the foundation of the hero's or heroine's journey as well as the path of initiation.

The late Paul Farmer warned that medical education could actually serve as "anesthesia for the young doctor's soul." He taught us that our primary allegiance is to the patient and that "science and technology will and should be the heart of modern medicine, but you must add the soul."[425] Common to all these medical activists is the message that medicine periodically loses its way. As doctors working in institutions with competing demands, we can lose our focus on what our primary responsibility is, and we can lose touch with our calling and our vows to heal and comfort the sick. In essence, we can lose our souls and medicine can lose its soul. How can we as individuals, and collectively as institutions, rediscover our souls?

Refounding as Institutional Soul Recovery

> By refounding I mean the process of returning to the founding experience of an organization or group in order to rediscover and re-own the vision and driving energy of the pioneers . . . I draw heavily on a model of initiation . . . of symbolic death and rebirth, which is made up of three stages—separation, transition/liminality and reaggregation.[426]
>
> GERALD ARBUCKLE

Gerald Arbuckle is a Catholic priest and anthropologist who has written extensively on the concept of refounding, whereby a "refounding person" takes on a leadership role to recapture the original vision of an institution, to revitalize it, and to bring it back into contemporary work life. We can think of refounding as soul recovery for institutions. Arbuckle has consulted widely with health care institutions, which he summarizes in his book *Humanizing Healthcare Reforms*. He describes five sub-cultural models in health care, including: 1) traditional (Indigenous), 2) foundational (humanitarian), 3) biomedical, 4) social, and 5) economic rationalist (business and management).[427] I found this very helpful, to view the tensions within contemporary medicine from the perspective of sub-cultural clashes of language and values.

Caring for self & others is a value of the traditional and foundational cultures of care. The social level is focused on population and public health, caring for society as a whole. The ascendancy of the biomedical culture and the economic rationalist cultures (documenting and billing) have often eclipsed the primary reason that health care organizations exist: to care for the suffering. Biomedical and economic rationalist cultures also share a love of numbers, counting, quantifying, and protocols. We need all these cultures to work together, but if we forget caring, we are no longer being healers, but rather technicians, protocol managers, and finance generators. While we need measurement-based care, we also need care-based care.

Many of the conflicts in health care stem from people speaking different "languages" and having values shaped by different cultural perspectives. Just as individuals can lose touch with their idealism and values through training and practice, institutions can lose sight of their visions and missions and become uncaring places where clinicians are still expected to care for patients without being cared for. Since caring is usually not quantified as an outcome measure, it can get lost in the data and process-improvement initiatives.

I met with Gerry Arbuckle in Australia in 2017 and had a long talk about some of these topics, followed by an email exchange, from which I offer a few of his comments about refounding.

> The initiation liminal experience of the refounding person is the transformative process of returning to the founding myth of an institution. He/she relives the founding experience in which the original founder was so shocked at the gap between their desired values and

> the realities of their world. The refounding person is alerted to the contemporary gap between values and the world around them. They are contemplatives who act; they move to bridge the gap, not by tackling the symptoms of the gap but by struggling to remove the *causes* of the gap. . . . Refounding persons commonly begin with a vague intuition of what should be done. By involving others in the planning and implementation of a project the refounding persons are slowly able to refine their insights and strategies. But collaborators cannot act *unless* they themselves experience the pain of the contemporary gap between values and realities, in imitation of the original founding pain.[428]

The refounding person goes through an initiation, experiencing the pain of the gap between the ideals of the institution and the contemporary state. The refounding person is a *contemplative who acts*, similar to Thich Nhat Hanh's concept of *engaged Buddhism*. As leaders, they are on their own journey. At some point this individual journey leads to inviting others who are suffering in the gap between the ideal and the actual to join them in the refounding journey. The idea of refounding brings together our focus on transformative learning, initiation, using suffering for growth, and the interplay of individual and institutional transformation.

If you find yourself *leading while exhausted*, doing refounding work may help you get your spark back and recover your healer's, educator's, or leader's soul. Personal refounding work takes you back to your own idealism and calling to go into your profession. When you become a refounding person, you expand beyond your own personal suffering to embrace the suffering of others and to work for transformation at cultural and institutional levels. I remember that when I took on the clinical director role at Buchanan Rehabilitation Centre in Auckland, New Zealand, I realized that part of the job was holding the suffering of staff. It can be "lonely at the top," because you have a broader perspective than individual employees and you are working at multiple different levels at the same time. One of the things I did as clinical director was to write a monthly newsletter, "Thoughts from the Clinical Director," where I would examine why we were doing this work, how healing happened, and how people who were lost could become found. I felt it was important to have a monthly reminder of the bigger picture of doing healing work in health care.

Whole Health & the Transformation of Health Care

It might seem like transforming health care is too big of a task, or too idealistic—but this is exactly what is happening in the Veterans Administration through the Office of Patient Centered Care & Cultural Transformation. Since 2011 this office has been working to transform health care to include a person-centered and holistic growth-centered model as well as a disease care model. (I have been working as a national education champion with this office since 2017, teaching VA staff across the country about Whole Health and self-care for themselves and for veterans). Research on the Whole Health model has shown benefits for veterans in decreasing opiate use and improved well-being, and for staff in lower burnout, lower turnover, and greater engagement and motivation.[429] A 2023 consensus report by the National Academies of Sciences, Engineering, and Medicine calls for whole health to be scaled and spread further throughout the VA and even into other health care delivery systems through the creation of a joint VA and Health and Human Services Center for Whole Health Innovation.

> Whole health is a common good that benefits people, families, and communities. Scaling and spreading whole health care so that all can have access to needed services is a tall task and will take seismic cultural, structural, and process transformations. These include but are not limited to how to think about what it means to be healthy, how to deliver health care, who is accountable for delivering health care, and even how to measure success.[430]

There is still a long way to go, but transformation of health care is possible! When I teach Whole Health, I focus on the fact that it applies equally to veterans as well as staff. We are all human beings and we can all work together to heal our own burnout, compassion fatigue, and soul loss, then we can all work together to heal and transform the system.

Repairing the World

> Some turn away from the work of repairing the world because of the pain of . . . alienation; others, because of the many discomforts, not all of them psychological, that are native to social justice work.[431]
>
> PAUL FARMER

We are here to do something and we are called to do something. We cannot just help ourselves; we have to help others, heal others, teach others, lead others. For some reason, that is just who we are—we are people who work with people. The world often seems so broken, people seem so broken, and in our work with people we become broken, too. It is okay. That is the first thing for us to understand—we are okay, but the world needs repairing. It is natural to periodically burst into a thousand pieces when you are in the line of work we are doing. Perhaps the goal is not to avoid becoming broken, but to learn how to break in such a way that we can, after a while, bring the pieces back together and deepen in our commitment to the work of *caring for self & others*, as Chenrezig did in the story that began the conversation of this book.

Here we will end with another story, remembering that all endings are just new beginnings. This story comes from Rachel Naomi Remen as told to Krista Tippett. The story came to Dr. Remen as her fourth birthday present from her grandfather.

> In the beginning there was only the holy darkness, the Ein Sof, the source of life. In the course of history, at a moment in time, this world, the world of a thousand thousand things, emerged from the heart of the holy darkness as a great ray of light. And then, perhaps because this is a Jewish story, there was an accident, and the vessels containing the light of the world, the

> wholeness of the world, broke. The wholeness of the world, the light of the world, was scattered into a thousand thousand fragments of light. And they fell into all events and all people, where they remain deeply hidden until this very day.
>
> Now, according to my grandfather, the whole human race is a response to this accident. We are here because we were born with the capacity to find the hidden light in all events and all people, to lift it up and make it visible once again and thereby restore the innate wholeness of the world. It's a very important story for our times. This task is called *tikkun olam* in Hebrew. It's the restoration of the world.
>
> And this is, of course, a collective task. It involves all people who have ever been born, all people presently alive, all people yet to be born. We are all healers of the world. That story opens a sense of possibility. It's not about healing the world by making a huge difference. It's about healing the world that touches you, that's around you.[432]

We start by healing our own souls—not some metaphysical abstraction, but that which is closest to us and makes us feel vital, alive, human. The ancients spoke of the World Soul, the *anima mundi*. They believed that we are all parts of the larger whole Soul. We are pieces of something larger than ourselves. As we gather together the shattered pieces of our selves, we gather together the shattered pieces of the Earth. With each individual repair we repair the world, we heal the Soul of the World. The repair of individuals and the repair of the world are not two different things—they are one.

LEADING CARING PRACTICE—CULTIVATING CARING

To lead caring, one must become caring. Caring is more than something we do, it is something that we are. We become the medicine that we need and then we give that medicine to others. This is not a technique, not a matter of *doing*, but more a matter of *being*—becoming a hollow bone and allowing caring to flow through us. This exercise is not something you are trying to do, but something that you are allowing to happen through you. Just as the heart functions through a balance of giving and receiving, so too leading caring is a state of being in which you are both giving and receiving.

This practice builds on the earlier loving-kindness meditation practice in chapter 4. You can use whatever word you wish that best describes the feeling of caring for you—loving-kindness, loving-careness, caring-ness, caring, or whatever best captures the feeling for you. Remember, this is not a mental practice about the idea of caring, but rather a cultivation of the feeling state of being caring.

Begin by finding a meditative posture. Take three deep, centering breaths. Recall the feeling of caring in your body when you imagine someone whom it is very easy to love. Picture this individual and notice what caring feels like in your body.

Now see if you can shift away from love for an individual to the feeling of love and caring itself. Notice whatever feelings and sensations arise.

Recall how the heart is constantly giving and receiving. Imagine caring flowing into and out of your heart, spreading throughout your body. Open to the heart of caring within yourself, and notice how caring is what the heart does. The heart is an ever-renewing and inexhaustible resource of caring. Allow this sense of caring to flow through you.

Imagine caring flowing from your heart into your left arm. Notice whatever feelings, sensations, or images arise as caring flows your left arm—color, temperature, vibration, openness, fullness, vitality—whatever form caring takes in your left arm, allow that experience to unfold from the center of your chest to the tips of your fingers. Notice your left arm filled with the vital aliveness of caring.

Imagine caring flowing from your heart into your right arm. Notice whatever feelings, sensations, or images accompany the experience of caring—color, temperature, vibration, openness, fullness, vitality—whatever form caring takes in your right arm, allow that experience to unfold from the center of your chest to the tips of your fingers. Notice your right arm filled with the vital aliveness of caring.

Imagine caring flowing from your heart down into your left leg. Notice whatever feelings, sensations, or images accompany the experience of caring as it flows down through your trunk, your left hip, your knee, your foot, and into the toes of your left foot. Notice your left leg filled with the vital aliveness of caring.

Imagine caring flowing from your heart down into your right leg. Notice whatever feelings, sensations, or images accompany the experience of caring as it flows down through your trunk, your right hip, your knee, your foot, and into the toes of your right foot. Notice your right leg filled with the vital aliveness of caring.

When you are ready, imagine caring flowing from your heart into your neck and head. Notice whatever feelings, sensations, or images accompany the experience of caring as it flows up into your head, gently washing over your brain, into your ears, eyes, nose, and mouth. Notice the experience of the vital aliveness of caring filling your head and neck.

Once you feel filled with caring, throughout your head and heart and body and arms and legs, take a few deep breaths, allowing caring to permeate your entire being. Once you are filled with caring, notice that caring might start to emanate, or pulsate, or flow outward from your body—caring flowing out your eyes, filling your mouth and flowing outward in your words, filling your hands and flowing outward to others whose lives you touch, and caring filling your feet and flowing outward, providing a pathway of caring for others who might follow in your footsteps.

The way to lead caring is to become caring. The way to become caring is to cultivate caring. The way to cultivate caring is to allow the flow of caring into and out of your heart, receiving and giving caring, giving and receiving caring. Allow caring to flow into you and out of you like a hollow bone. Allow your heart to give and receive and receive and give caring, replenishing caring throughout your body and being. Allow the vision of your eyes to see with caring. Allow your ears to open and listen with caring. Allow your mouth to be filled with caring and to speak words of caring to others. Allow your hands to be filled with caring so that every life you touch is touched by caring. Allow your feet to be filled with caring so that every step you take is in harmony with caring and creates a pathway of caring for others who might follow you.

Joseph Rael likes to say, "What comes around goes around," and "We are the People of the Circle." He tells us, "If you take care of Mother Earth, she will take care of you." So walk with caring on Mother Earth and create pathways of caring through your life, through your actions, and through your words, and you will be cared for as you care for others.

Conclusion

THE FULL CIRCLE OF CARING

IN THE BEGINNING of the book, I introduced the metaphor of health care as a jet plane with a gaping hole sucking out all the oxygen. In such a situation you need to put on your own oxygen mask first—you need to care for self before caring for others. Hopefully this book has given you numerous ideas and practices for putting on your own oxygen mask and *breathing in caring.*

The next step is *breathing out caring*—caring for others, helping others to put on their oxygen masks, and addressing their wounds and their suffering.

There is a third aspect of addressing the caring and compassion crisis in health care: repairing the hole in the fuselage to stop the loss of oxygen we are all experiencing. At this level, caring for self and caring for others is the same thing because we are all in this together.

Each of these different levels—self, other, system—are challenges that require a different focus and yet all are about the same thing: *caring.* Caring cannot be something that just happens between health care workers and clients or patients. Caring has to be the foundation of the system and the basis of every interaction within the system—between staff and patients, between staff and staff, and between leadership and staff. Caring is the oxygen that allows us to do our work. It may not be visible when it is present, but when it is absent everyone suffers. We can think of the compassion crisis in health care, and so many other fields, not as an individual problem with individual solutions, but as a systemic and institutional problem that affects us all. The costs of caring—burnout, compassion fatigue, soul loss, and others—are not simply too much caring going out from the health care worker, but also a deficit of care for workers, and a lack of caring in the clinical atmosphere. The dilemma is, how do we change the system when we are only individuals?

Parker Palmer writes that "institutions *are* us."[433] Institutions are made up of individuals, so transformation at the individual level can lead to system change. When we embark on a post-burnout growth journey of transforming our self, we create a *glowing* node of caring within the institution. The more people who become glowing nodes of caring in a system, the brighter and more filled with caring the system becomes. Conversely, the more people who burn out, fall into compassion fatigue, and lose connection with their souls, the more *glooming* nodes proliferate within the system. Glooming can range from a dimmed light of caring to actually giving off darkness, heaviness, and cynicism that sucks the light of caring, the oxygen of caring, out of the system. We are all in this together. To only save your ego is to lose the self—and the system needs each one of us, glowing and giving off compassion, if health care is to be truly caring.

Obviously, leaders and managers have more influence on the glooming or glowing of the atmosphere of caring within a system, and yet leaders and managers are individuals, too. If a leader's self is glooming, it can bring down the whole team or institution. A leader's responsibility is to nurture the caring atmosphere of the team. If leaders do the work of caring for self, they can become beacons of glowing caring for the systems they work in. This can make it easier for team members to care for themselves as well as for others. Caring is the essence of compassionate humanity that fuels healthy work environments.

DEVELOPING A PRACTICE FOR POST-BURNOUT GROWTH

> Medicine, like yoga, like the entirety of this existence on earth, is a daily practice. It is the opportunity, should we choose it, to heal the human body and spirit. By healing ourselves, we heal each other. By healing each other, we heal ourselves.[434]
>
> MICHELE HARPER

As the quote by Dr. Harper states, medicine and yoga are both daily practices that heal and bring us together. Sometimes the narrative around self-care for health care workers has a shaming and blaming aspect, that if we took better care of ourselves we would not suffer the costs of caring. We need to shift our idea of self-care practices from another productivity measure we do for external reasons to practices that are internally motivated because they nurture the joy of living.

I've been thinking a lot about the idea of a yoga of burnout, a daily and weekly practice of working with suffering and finding joy in my life.[435] The word "yoga" comes from the Sanskrit, meaning "union, yoking."[436] We can think of a yoga practice as not just a series of physical postures on a mat, but as an ongoing practice of bringing back together (yoking and unifying) the fragmented pieces of ourselves. This is, then, a continuing human education practice to care for ourselves and to nurture our full humanity. Yoga, as originally described in Patanjali's *Yoga Sutras*, included both meditation and physical postures, as well as a series of practices for developing our full humanity. We can think of a yoga of burnout in this broader way of bringing together mind and body, body and spirit, ego and Self, as well as self and other—bringing together, healing, whatever has been separated or fragmented.

Poet and teacher Mark Nepo has written about this kind of idea of unifying practice in his book *The Endless Practice: Becoming Who You Were Born to Be.* At first, the idea of endless practice could be overwhelming or depressing, but Nepo points out that we are always breathing and our heart is always beating and those are the kind of practices he wants to emphasize.

> The tasks are endless. The wonder is endless. The pain of living is endless. The chances to love are endless. In actuality, living is an endless practice, through which we become who we were born to be, step-by-step, face-to-face, heart-to-heart. . . . No matter how hard we work, the aim and purpose of practice is not to be done with it, but to immerse ourselves so completely in life by any means that we, for the moment, are life living itself. Excellence, if we achieve it, is a welcome by-product of complete immersion. But the reward for practice is a thoroughness of being.[437]

Practice, then, is its own reward in cultivating "thoroughness of being," or we could say fully human being, or we could say reconnecting with our souls. Practice is not to prevent burnout, but to practice being human. Practice is not to prevent suffering, but to accept it and use it as part of the larger project of becoming who we are.

Yogi Stephen Cope has written about the Sanskrit word *samvega*: "a complex state involving a kind of disillusionment with mundane life, and a wholehearted longing for a deeper investigation into the inner workings of the mind and self."[438] This reminds me of burnout and soul loss, as well as of Mezirow's disorienting dilemma that initiates transformational learning. A yoga practitioner would see burnout/*samvega* as a gift that brings "an unshakeable resolve to develop as a fully alive human being."[439]

Burnout, compassion fatigue, soul loss—the costs of caring—are complex states, like *samvega*. They involve disillusionment, a longing for wholeness, and a quest for the soul, reanimating us as full human beings. In this way, burnout, compassion fatigue, and soul loss can serve as an invitation to initiation to transform suffering.

In her book *The Joy of Burnout: How the End of the World Can Be a New Beginning*, Dina Glouberman writes that the suffering of burnout can be a hidden message that can lead us to joy. From a transformational perspective, she states that "rather than being cured, burnout needs to be honoured and listened to."[440] We don't want to "get rid of" burnout, we want to learn from it. According to Glouberman, burnout is a gift that invites us to attend to our inner being so that we can create a good home for the soul. She writes, "If we create a beautiful home for the soul, the soul will naturally create a beautiful life for us and for others. . . . Joy is the free gift of the soul. It is literally the love of our life."[441] Burnout can be a call for us to shift our focus from the external world to our inner world, to do some inner house cleaning, and see how we can make our interior lives beautiful and inviting for the soul to return.

In working with soul loss, we become healers of the soul. The Greek word for soul is *psyche* and the word for healer or physician is *iatros*. Combining the two gives us *psyche-iatros*—in the old words, a healer of the soul. Burnout invites us all, regardless of our education and qualifications, to become a kind of *psychiatros*—a healer of the soul who seeks to bring together the fragmented and lost pieces of ourselves, integrating together into a greater whole as a wounded healer. In the tradition of the concept of the *anima mundi*, the soul of the world, we are all called to heal our own souls as well as that of the world when we are soul sick or have lost our souls. We shouldn't leave soul healing just to psychiatrists, many of whom have abandoned the soul and have become technicians managing brain chemicals.

My idea of a yoga of burnout is a daily and weekly practice of yoking together the fragmented pieces of our selves and souls. You can call this practice whatever best suits you. For me, calling it a yoga practice reminds me that it is an ongoing practice, endless as Mark Nepo reminds us—a way of living and being, a way of caring for humanity, our own and others.

FINDING MENTORS & RITUAL ELDERS TO RE-MEMBER OUR SELVES

Let's return to the story of Chenrezig. The first half of the story is a typical health care worker tragedy of burnout—an individual tries to care for others and ends up becoming wounded themselves, bursting into a thousand pieces. Unfortunately, this story is repeated in different variations on a daily basis, across the world—not just in health care, but in education, business, even parenting, and in any kind of environment where caring for others occurs. Well-intentioned leaders encourage the Chenrezigs of the world to take a little time off, to engage in self-care, to build up their resilience, and get themselves back in the game so that they can be productive and efficient work units. This model is not working. Heroic self-care, outside work hours by the individual alone, is not the solution. Without systemic change self-care is only a bandage. It is like telling workers that they should do breathing exercises after work so that they can hold their breath longer when they come back to work in an oxygen/caring-deprived occupational environment.

How does Chenrezig transform? In the narrative, transformation requires what Robert Moore calls "ritual elders," someone who has passed through their own struggles and has a bigger perspective of wisdom and compassion to support post-burnout growth in others. Even buddhas sometimes need buddhas of compassion like Amitābha.

The ritual elder could be someone in a formal leadership role, a senior member of the team, or sometimes even better, someone outside the team hierarchy who can serve as a mentor. This is the way that human beings have practiced transformation throughout the ages. "Mentor" was originally the name of the elder who counseled Odysseus' son, Telemachus, while Odysseus was away ten years fighting in the war described in the *Iliad* and the additional ten years journeying home in the *Odyssey*. The goddess Athena would use Mentor as a vehicle (a hollow bone) to speak to Telemachus to support him with divine wisdom when he was thrust into the political world at a young age.

The mentor doesn't have to know everything; Athena, or we could say wise inspiration, can come through the mentor when they enter into a ritual elder role. Our word "mentor" has come to mean "wise adviser, intimate friend, who also is a sage counselor,"[442] and it is this caring function that is so often missing in work settings and the contemporary world. When an individual is disoriented and hurting, we need someone from the work community to take the *time* to create the *space* and provide the *support* that the sufferer needs to heal. These three things that are one thing (*time-space-support*) create the ecosystem of caring.

The story of Chenrezig teaches that we can grow beyond our previous limitations, but this may require a mentor or ritual elder to provide time-space-support. The caring attention, mentorship, and initiation that Amitābha gives allows Chenrezig to grow beyond his previous ability to care—instead of two eyes, Chenrezig now has a thousand eyes; instead of two arms, now he has a thousand arms. Chenrezig is not only better able to see and touch the suffering of others, he also can now serve as a ritual elder for the next generation of wounded healers. The full circle of healing means that what one receives, one will eventually give to others.

What is the metaphorical meaning of having a thousand eyes and a thousand arms? Perhaps it is developing a new way of seeing suffering in addition to being a technician. Maybe it is the wisdom of seeing suffering as intrinsic to human life and that all of us, health care workers and patients alike, are vulnerable to suffering. Maybe it is seeing that to give compassion and caring to another can be a small spark in the compassion revolution, creating a ripple effect of a little less glooming and a little more glowing of caring in the world. Maybe having a thousand eyes and a thousand arms is a metaphor for a shift from head to heart, in which the eyes and powers of the heart are opened and activated. When the eyes of the heart are opened, we become caring in our very being—even while performing technical interventions. Rather than seeing caring as something that occurs through a sack of tools we carry and manipulate, maybe caring is something that carries us through our challenging days. The transformation that Chenrezig undergoes allows him to be a healer for self as well as others—a transformation that situates him in the position of a wise elder who can re-member other healers in turn.

As Joseph Rael tells us, within the medicine bag of our hearts we have sacred medicines. Perhaps the solution to burnout, compassion fatigue, and soul loss is dormant within each of us, the held-back goodness[443] within the medicine bags of our hearts. The solution is not something we need to do, but something we must become. Even that is not quite correct, because caring is already within us—caring is in you, caring is in me, caring is in us.

As Amitābha did for Chenrezig (and Beautiful Painted Arrow did for me), a ritual elder and mentor reawakens our hearts so that we can reconnect with our held-back goodness, re-member and remember our healing vows, and remember who we are as healers. An elder and a mentor's role is to help us become who we are, not necessarily to make us well-adjusted, productive, and efficient work units.

BECOMING WOUNDED HEALERS & WOUNDED STORYTELLERS

Our challenge is to transform the wound into wisdom and compassion. It is a difficult journey from being wounded to becoming wounded healers. By becoming wounded storytellers, we can change our narratives from being victims to having something to give to ourselves and others—healing and caring. In his book *The Wounded Storyteller*, Arthur Frank writes about possible narratives that one can have when going through an illness experience: the *restitution narrative* (trying to get back to how things were), the *chaos narrative* (being lost in fragmentation), and the *quest narrative* (putting the pieces back together again and creating a new narrative). Much of the focus on burnout takes the form of the restitution narrative—trying, through self-care and resilience, to get back to how things were before burnout, compassion fatigue, and soul loss. Frank's description of the quest narrative is more similar to the transformational approach of post-burnout growth we are focusing on in *Caring for Self & Others*. Within the quest narrative, Frank writes that there are three elements: memoir, manifesto, and automythology. *Memoir* is often in the form of an "interrupted autobiography."[444] The *manifesto* "asserts that illness is a social issue, not simply a personal affliction."[445] The third element or path Frank describes is *automythology*.

> Automythology fashions the author as one who not only has survived, but has been reborn. Like the manifesto, the automythology reaches out, but its language is more personal than political. Individual change, not social reform, is emphasized, with the author as an exemplar of this change. . . . Automythology turns the specific illness into a paradigm of universal conflicts and concerns. The body of the storyteller becomes a pivot point between microcosm and macrocosm.[446]

We can all think of ourselves as wounded storytellers, just as Chenrezig's story of wounding leads through fragmentation (chaos), to memoir (reviewing his wounded healer narrative), to manifesto (changing the world for the better), and then elaborating his automythology (renewing his vow to alleviate suffering that incorporates his memoir). The concept of automythology might seem a bit strange if you think of mythology as something make-believe; however if you think of it as a form of active, creative imagination, it can be a way that you develop your own story by exploring your calling.

In the mythology of Chenrezig, his tears became supportive inner goddesses, his suffering is valuable and recognized by a buddha of compassion, and his fragmentation into a thousand pieces becomes a gift and a strength of having a thousand eyes and a thousand arms.

How might you work with the details of your own narrative—remembering your vow and calling, tracing your path that lead to your wounding and fragmentation, how you have found inner and outer helpers and supports, and how you have found transformation in your life, bringing healing to yourself and others? How might you put together the fragmented pieces of your soul and self to create a healing narrative of your life and work? Try journaling on these questions as an automythology practice.

Our challenge is to create our own stories of transformation, our own stories of post-burnout growth, from the fragments of our own lives. We do this by working with our suffering, acknowledging the role of suffering in transformation, and by supporting each other in finding our voices as wounded healers and wounded storytellers. Maybe we can even go beyond the wound (as wounding is one of the things that makes us human), becoming healed healers and healed storytellers.

Epilogue

CANCER & BEYOND

> **patient (adj.)** *paciente*, "capable of enduring misfortune, suffering, etc., without complaint"... from Latin *patientem* "bearing, supporting, suffering, enduring, permitting"...
>
> **patient (n.)** "suffering, injured, or sick person under medical treatment"[447]

BECOMING A PATIENT can be an education for a doctor, at least that is how I try to look at it. It is such a different view from inside the medical system as a patient than as a doctor. There is so much suffering within the medical system—the most obvious being that of the patient, but there is also the suffering of the staff from the costs of caring.

When I was diagnosed with nevoid melanoma in August of 2022, I geared up for some serious self-care. I felt I had been training my whole life for a self-care marathon, and after the initial shock, I felt I was up for it. Steven Wang's *Beating Melanoma* describes two phases of cancer treatment: the "mad rush" phase (initial diagnosis, rapid-fire scans, and evaluations) and the "marathon" phase (ongoing treatment, long-term side effects, worries about recurrence).[448] I found this distinction helpful as I felt an initial adrenaline rush, rapidly assimilating information and coming to terms with the medical system in the mad rush phase, and then shifting to the long-term perspective of living day-by-day with symptoms, side effects, screenings, and treatment.

Leading up to my surgery, I focused on supporting myself in all the Ten Dimensions of Being Fully Human as described in this book. I adapted my *yoga of burnout* to a *yoga of cancer* program and made a weekly grid to chart my practices. I sought to balance working with my pain and suffering with cultivating joy and bliss. It felt supportive to make more time for these practices in my life rather than putting them off until I could get to them. I tried to do what I love first. I went into surgery with a good attitude and a can-do mindset.

In October 2022, I had a wide-excision of the melanoma in my left upper arm along with a sentinel node biopsy of two lymph nodes in my left axilla (armpit). Both nodes showed local spread of melanoma, yielding a cancer staging of IIIa. I had a side effect of lymphatic cording, in which lymphatic vessels become fibrotic or scarred after damage from the surgery. I had a palpable cord running from my shoulder to my elbow and I even sometimes had pain or discomfort down into my wrist and fingers. I started physical therapy (PT), but months after surgery I still have occasional discomfort.

Around the time of starting PT, I was missing a big chunk of my left arm, I had two large scars, and the cording limited my daily exercise and yoga. My "quick recovery from cancer" narrative was interrupted. I started to struggle more to keep positive. I read somewhere that cancer and melancholia were both thought to be disorders of black bile (*melaina chole*) in the humoral theory that was prevalent from the time of Hippocrates up into the 1700–1800s. I found this interesting and looked at the linguistic similarities of "melanoma" and "melancholia," and my reading turned to memoirs of cancer, doctors writing on cancer and the new science of immunotherapy (with optimistic talk of finding the cure for cancer), and writings on melancholia.

I met with my oncologist to discuss options for adjuvant treatment to prevent recurrence and he recommended immunotherapy.

The way he saw it, I had around an 80% five-year survival rate without further treatment, but with immunotherapy that might increase to around 90%. However, my reading about this relatively new treatment of immunotherapy was that there was about a 10% chance that I could develop a potentially permanent side effect. I was particularly concerned about my family history of rheumatoid arthritis in my maternal grandmother, first cousin, and her daughter.

On the one hand, the numbers seemed to mean everything. I went round and round trying to have the numbers make the decision of whether to start immunotherapy for me. On the other hand, the numbers were meaningless on an individual level, as I would either get side effects or not. I would either live or die—I couldn't be 80% alive. The other thing with these numbers was that when I told people I had an 80–90% five-year survival rate, many would feel relieved and say, "That is good news!" Maybe in a game that is good news, but if you look at it as having a 10–20% chance of not being alive in five years, no one would say "That is good news!" Eventually, I decided to go on a yearlong immunotherapy protocol with monthly infusions.

Let me tell you, when an oncologist describes "mild side effects," their reference point is death! On immunotherapy, a good day felt like I was *recovering* from the flu, and a bad day felt like I was *coming down* with the flu. During the treatment, I have felt continually lousy with malaise, muscle aches, and fatigue. I was able to work through the body aches, malaise, and headaches, feeling somewhere between unwell and not good.

The real problem, however, was something else. About two weeks after my first infusion I developed neuropathy symptoms on the bottom of my right foot. My oncologist's reaction felt dismissive, saying somewhat incredulously that there was a less than 1% chance of that side effect on this medicine. Over time the tingling sensation spread to my left foot as well. Then, two weeks after my third infusion, the neuropathy took off like wildfire, spreading from the bottoms of my feet to my chest in less than two weeks. I ended up in the emergency department twice, and I was started on a high dose of oral steroids to shut off my hyped-up immune system from the immunotherapy. This halted the upward progression of the symptoms, keeping them below the waist.

However, the steroids had a number of side effects—interfering with sleep, increasing tremor and clumsiness, feeling very hyped up, and worsening cognitive symptoms.

When I started tapering down on the steroids, the neuropathy symptoms started to ascend up my body again, although at a slower pace. When I was on about half the dose of steroids, the symptoms reached my chest and back, and when I was almost off the steroid, the symptoms of tingling, burning sensations, electric jolts, and cramping pain reached my neck, face, and scalp. I've since lost the hair on parts of my legs. The aching took root in the muscles to the degree that a rheumatologist thought it was consistent with polymyalgia rheumatica and I've started on a course of low-dose steroids. The prototypical neuropathy symptoms of electric jolts and burning pain have given way to a continuous feeling of an inner tremor or inner vibration throughout my body.

NARRATIVE WRECKAGE: LOST IN THE WILDERNESS OF THE BODY

Arthur Frank describes how illness can cause a "narrative wreckage," as the "illness story begins in wreckage, having lost its map and destination. The story is both interrupted and about interruption."[449] I have acutely felt this sense of wreckage and loss of orientation at many different points in my cancer experience, but most profoundly when I had rapidly ascending neurological symptoms and I felt like the medical team (other than an amazing oncology nurse and dermatologist) was always a couple of steps behind and didn't seem to grasp how fast the symptoms were moving and how potentially life-threatening they could become. Also, I felt I was falling between the cracks of the medical institutional framework that reductively divides people up into different specialties for different organ systems. Even though my symptoms were affecting my whole body, I was referred to many providers who would focus on only a part of me: surgical oncology, medical oncology, neurology, rheumatology, dermatology, emergency medicine, physical therapists, dieticians, integrative medicine, functional medicine, and primary care. I felt like the proverbial elephant being diagnosed by the blind men: everyone saw a piece of the puzzle, but no one had the whole picture—except maybe my acupuncturist.

I often felt that I was lost within the wilderness of the body. Rather than my body being a way of being in the world and interacting with the world, my focus was involuntarily limited to the functioning of my body. Cognitive dulling and slowing made it more challenging to socialize. It felt like I could see people through the trees on the wilderness' edge, but the trees were often thick and sometimes I could only glimpse the outside world. Fatigue and pain symptoms also trapped me in the wilderness of the body, making it difficult to do the most basic things.

When I spoke with Joseph Rael about the melanoma and treatment, he could relate—he himself had melanoma a few years earlier and went through immunotherapy and had some similar side effects. He asked me why I thought I had cancer, but before I could answer he blurted out, "Because you are still in training!" I tried to adopt this attitude of being in training, of having the opportunity to learn something. I started to explore the inner wilderness. I tried to learn what I could about illness and being a patient. I embraced melanoma and melancholia as my teachers and I even try to meditate on the inner tremor as a manifestation of *spanda*, the divine creative pulsation.

I tried to be both a good patient and a good doctor—making summaries and timelines of my symptoms, researching possible causes and immunotherapy complications, and reporting my rapidly evolving symptoms. In the end I came to feel that I was a burden and a puzzle and that I couldn't get basic questions answered satisfactorily—why was my copper level low, why was I having gait abnormalities, why was my balance off? I was not only trying to make sense of what I was going through, creating some meaningful narrative, but I was also trying to find the medical narrative that could lead to appropriate evaluations and treatment. I needed my medical team to be there with me, to be concerned about the breakneck speed of the symptoms, and to admit when they didn't know something instead of clinging to some medical lingo factoid that didn't really answer my questions and felt invalidating. I needed my medical team to enter into the wilderness I was lost in, not just to make pronouncements and benedictions from outside the forest. The more I tried to communicate and elaborate the swift-changing symptoms, the more isolated I felt. At one point I felt like I was drowning in quicksand and that my team was waving at me from solid ground, encouraging me to wait for treatment until they could figure out what kind of sand I was drowning in. I felt alone, scared, frustrated, depressed, and angry.

At first, when I told people I had cancer, they would say, "I'm sorry you are sick." It was funny; I didn't feel sick, that really wasn't what I was going through. It was only later, with the immunotherapy (after having no evident cancer), that I first started feeling sick. It was tolerable most of the time. Once the neuropathy symptoms caught fire, though, I couldn't work and felt bad all the time. I couldn't keep up with charting my practices during the week for my yoga of cancer program. At times I could only re-read science fiction novels on the sofa and really couldn't give a dang about any self-care programs. I realized that I needed to add another practice—a practice of doing nothing! At the worst point, even with a cane I couldn't walk more than a couple blocks, and that was a continuous effort. Even to simply stand upright was a strain on my thighs and low back.

When I was on prednisone, I could only sleep two to three hours at a time, maybe four hours tops, and then I would be up for an hour or two. I was reading books on yoga in the middle of the night and started practicing yoga and meditation during these times. I decided I might as well enroll in an online yoga teacher certification training and work toward some goal. I'm still not sure if that was a good idea or not. On the one hand, it is something I have always wanted to do. I could usually manage an hour of watching a yoga teaching video and thirty to sixty minutes of yoga on the mat, and it gave me a new focus for my self-care rehabilitation program. On the other hand, it created a feeling of always needing to be productive and working on the training rather than just napping and reading on the sofa—doing "nothing."

I share all this with you to reflect on the many challenges of self-care and also the ways in which we can turn self-care into another productivity protocol. Also, I share my own experience with illness and the medical system to remind us of all the challenges that patients face and the ways that our medical institutions can invalidate and marginalize human beings.

My cancer and complications with treatment came on the heels of a pandemic, the shift to tele-work and tele-medicine, politicization of public health, growing polarization in culture and politics, racism, social justice issues, war, and climate crisis. During the past few years I have also struggled with being at odds with the treatment philosophy of my clinical service. I've felt invalidated through the university for my scholarly activities and book publications not being "academic" enough, and even found myself doubting whether I had anything to offer students and patients. This has been a time of constant uncertainty and continuous adaptation and re-adaptation. It is not only too much in one arena, it is *too-much-too-much*—too many things that are too much. Sometimes, as I was working on this book, I have felt at a loss for how to talk about clinician well-being in the face of all this. Well-being seems like too lofty of a goal. A meditation teacher, Sam Voolstra, suggested to me that "okay-ness" is a more reasonable goal.[450] I have had days where it takes all my energy just to reach okay, but it is far more attainable than the goal of flourishing well-being!

All this is life. I don't mean this to complain; I try to be patient—as doctors and health care professionals, we have to have to be patient, too. As the etymology of the word "patient" reminds us, we have to be "capable of enduring misfortune, suffering, etc., without complaint."

Our own struggles can seem small when compared to the ravages of war and cultural clashes of history. And yet, our suffering is our own and if we do not work skillfully with it, it can poison us, robbing us of our idealism and leaving us demoralized and cynical.

In my own practice of caring for self & others, I try to maintain hope. Without hope, I stop caring and fall off my practices. I also notice times that I approach my practices as if they were another performance measure I was trying to meet. At these times I give myself permission to take a break, to do nothing for a while, and then I re-evaluate. The essence of caring is love and nurturing, and we all need to be careful that we don't set up systems or practices that run on something other than love.

Caring is a continuous practice. As we go through life, our narratives need constant repair and attention because we are always evolving into the unknown. Burnout, compassion fatigue, soul loss—the costs of caring—can cause us to lose the thread of our narrative, and we become lost in the wilderness. Arthur Frank and Chenrezig remind us that we can always refashion our narrative, embarking on a quest to heal ourselves and bring together the fragmented pieces of our lives.

It can be daunting and demoralizing to try to care for self, let alone others, when there is so much uncaring in systems and the world. We don't have to do it alone. We can cultivate communities of caring that support us as individuals and help us take on the work of transforming systems. I will give an example of two transformational systems I work with that replenish hope for me.

Jonathan McFarland created the international Doctor as a Humanist (DASH) organization in 2017. He has brought together an idealistic medical humanities team from around the globe, and is "bringing back the heart and soul to medicine." I started speaking at DASH events and am now on the steering committee. Jonathan has become a great friend. We speak often, sharing our KU and MU levels for the day (Kopacz Units and McFarland Units), reflecting on the journey of illness, and providing mutual support to each other.

Closer to home, I have a one-day-per-week position with the VA's national Office of Patient Centered Care & Cultural Transformation (OPCC&CT). In this role I develop and revise curricula and teach courses to VA staff across the country, such as "Taking Time to Care" and "Whole Health for Well-Being." In our courses we teach staff to use Whole Health to care for themselves so that they can use Whole Health to support veterans. We are working to transform the culture of the VA, the largest integrated health care system in the United States. My work with *Re-humanizing Medicine* preceded my time at the VA, however there is substantial overlap between the dimensions of being fully human and the VA Whole Health framework's focus on mind, body, relationships, surroundings, and spirit and soul. An abundance of Whole Health materials are available online that are open access to veterans and the public.[451] Even better than the organization of OPCC&CT are the people who work for it. Many of my best friends at the VA are not at my local facility, but are spread throughout the country. Compassionate, committed, creative—this group of healers continually inspires me.

In addition to the two mentioned here, many other organizations around the world are working on what I call the compassion revolution. Find one or start one to get the support you need. Systems and institutions were created by individuals and we, as individuals, are the life-blood, the heart and soul of institutions. Let's all put on our oxygen masks, take a breath, attend to those around us, and start to transform the systems we work in.

ACKNOWLEDGMENTS

FIRST AND FOREMOST, I want to thank Laura Merritt for working on earlier versions of this book and providing developmental editing, caring, and companionship.

Thanks to Shelly Francis, editor and publisher at Creative Courage Press, for her caring and attention to detail, making this a better book. Thank you to Rebecca Job for her editing work on the words and skeletal structure of this book.

Julia Yates—gratitude for her feedback as a reader of the text and for the joy of teaching Whole Health Well-Being together.

Thank you to my entire medical team for their work to restore my body to health. Particular thanks to Andrew Szalay for his steady guidance, Nurse Sunny for her ever-present support, and to Anna Cogen who seamlessly integrates the roles of healer and technician while proving that healing is more than skin deep. A special thank you to my acupuncturist, Mark Tibeau, for his unwavering support, sense of humor, and for accompanying me into the wilderness of the body.

Thank you to my VA colleagues: Brad Felker, mentor, colleague, friend—whose support and humor is a lifeline; DJ Nurse Jenny Salmon for her deep caring work; Kori Blitstein for her support during my illness; and my friend and colleague Eileen Bennhoff for her comments on the text—I am honored to work alongside such a healer! Thanks to

Sadie Elisseou for her feedback on grounding and trauma-informed care and to Lori Katz for her optimism, clinical work, and writing. Thank you to Mike Lee, Ceremonial Elder of the VA Sweat Lodge at American Lake VA, for his teaching and support. A big thanks to Lucy Houghton for doing and discussing post-burnout growth. Lastly, to Steve Hunt for all the Daweed-ing and Stephen-ing that surely makes the world a better place.

Appreciation to past and present Whole Health Education Champions (WHEC) and healers from the VA Office of Patient Centered Care—particularly Carol Bowman, Stephanie Brown-Johnson, Marité Hagman, Michael Hollifield, Jen McDonald, Yani Nieves, Adam Rindfleisch, Henri Roca, Aysha Saeed, Codi Schale, Greg Serpa, Tulika Singh, trickster Chris Smith, Kerri Weishoff, Prachi Garodia, and all the rest—they are all true healers and caretakers of caring and transformation! Another WHEC deserves additional recognition—Carlann Defontes, for her friendship, her hospitality, and for walking beside me as another healer on a path of healing.

Thank you to Jonathan McFarland, president of The Doctor as a Humanist and all the wonderful healers involved with that organization, and Javier de la Maza of Ars Medica. Jonathan, may your MU (McFarland Units) continue to trend ever upwards!

Last but not least, thank you to my family. Thank you to my wife, Mary Pat, for her continual caring and support on this long, strange trip of life through sickness and in health. My parents, Tom and Linda Kopacz, thanks for their caring for all the lost and wounded plants and animals—including me and my sister! My sister, Karen Kopacz, thank you for all the collaborations on projects and technical support and design for my website and blog.

Blessings to Joseph Rael (Beautiful Painted Arrow) for opening your heart and sharing the vastness of who you are.

ENDNOTES

1 This is my paraphrase from Bokar Rinpoche, *Chenrezig, Lord of Love* (San Francisco: ClearPoint Press, 1991), 28–33.

2 Pamela Gayle White, "Taking Care of Others (Without Exploding into a Thousand Bits): Timely advice for countering burnout," *Tricycle*, March 28, 2021, https://tricycle.org/article/burnout/.

3 David R. Kopacz and J. Greg Serpa, "Clinician Resilience," in *Integrative Medicine*, 5th ed., ed. David Rakel and Vincent Minichiello (Philadelphia: Elsevier, 2022), 33.

4 David Kopacz, "Beyond Resilience: Fighting the Causes of the Burnout Pandemic," CLOSLER: Moving Us Closer to Osler, A Miller Coulson Academy of Clinical Excellence Initiative, Johns Hopkins Medicine, November 3, 2020, https://closler.org/lifelong-learning-in-clinical-excellence/beyond-resilience-fighting-the-causes-of-the-burnout-pandemic.

5 Cheryl S. Al-Mateen et al., "Vicarious Traumatization and Coping in Medical Students: A Pilot Study," *Academic Psychiatry* 39 (2015): 90–93, https://doi.org/10.1007/s40596-014-0199-3.

6 Debra Klamen, Linda Grossman, and David Kopacz, "Posttraumatic Stress Disorder Symptoms in Resident Physicians Related to Their Internship," *Academic Psychiatry* 19 (1995): 142–49, https://doi.org/10.1007/BF03341425.

7 David Kopacz, *Re-humanizing Medicine: A Holistic Framework for Transforming Your Self, Your Practice, and the Culture of Medicine* (Washington DC: Ayni Books, 2014).

8 Omar Sultan Haque and Adam Waytz, "Dehumanization in Medicine: Causes, Solutions, and Functions," *Perspectives on Psychological Science* 7, no. 2 (2012): 176–86, https://doi.org/10.1177/1745691611429706.

9 Stewart Gabel, "Demoralization in Health Professional Practice: Development, Amelioration, and Implications for Continuing Education," *Journal of Continuing Education in the Health Professions* 33, no. 2 (Spring 2013): 118–26, https://doi.org/10.1002/chp.21175.

10 Mark Linzer, Elizabeth Griffiths, and Mitchell Feldman, "Responding to the Great Resignation: Detoxify and Rebuild the Culture," *Journal of General Internal Medicine* 37 (December 2022): 4276–77, https://doi.org/10.1007/s11606–022-07703–1.

11 Cynda Hylton Rushton, *Moral Resilience: Transforming Moral Suffering in Healthcare* (New York: Oxford University Press, 2018).

12 Victor Dzau, Darrell Kirch, and Thomas Nasca, "To Care Is Human—Collectively Confronting the Clinician-Burnout Crisis," *New England Journal of Medicine* 378, no. 4 (January 25, 2018): 312–14, https://doi.org/10.1056/NEJMp1715127.

13 Ying-Ying Zhang et al., "Extent of compassion satisfaction, compassion fatigue and burnout in nursing: A meta-analysis," *Journal of Nursing Management* 26, no. 7 (October 2018): 810–19, https://doi.org/10.1111/jonm.12589.

14 Hannah McCormack et al., "The prevalence and cause(s) of burnout among applied psychologists: A systematic review," *Frontiers in Psychology* 16, no. 9 (October 2018), https://doi.org/10.3389/fpsyg.2018.01897.

15 Gabrielle Simionato and Susan Simpson, "Personal risk factors associated with burnout among psychotherapists: A systematic review of the literature," *Journal of Clinical Psycholo*gy 74, no. 9 (September 2018): 1431–56, https://doi.org/10.1002/jclp.22615.

16 Eric Jotkoff, "NEA survey: Massive staff shortages in schools leading to educator burnout; alarming number of educators indicating they plan to leave profession," National Education Association, February 1, 2022, https://www.nea.org/about-nea/media-center/press-releases/nea-survey-massive-staff-shortages-schools-leading-educator.

17 Jim Harter, "Manager Burnout Is Only Getting Worse," Gallup, November 18, 2021, accessed August 2, 2022, https://www.gallup.com/workplace/357404/manager-burnout-getting-worse.aspx.

18 "Women leaders continue to feel the burn of burnout," McKinsey and Company website, February 2, 2022, https://www.mckinsey.com/featured-insights/coronavirus-leading-through-the-crisis/charting-the-path-to-the-next-normal/women-leaders-continue-to-feel-the-burn-of-burnout.

19 Luca Morgantini et al., "Factors contributing to healthcare professional burnout during the COVID-19 pandemic: A rapid turnaround global survey," *PLOS ONE* 15, no. 9 (September 3, 2020): e0238217, https://doi.org/10.1371/journal.pone.0238217.

20 Herbert Freudenberger, "Staff Burn-Out," *Journal of Social Issues* 30, no. 1 (Winter 1974): 159–65.

21 Christina Maslach and Michael Leiter, "Understanding the burnout experience: recent research and its implications for psychiatry," *World Psychiatry* 15, no. 2 (June 2016): 103–11, https://doi.org/10.1002/wps.20311.

22 Christina Maslach, "An interview with Christina Maslach," interview by Gail Kinman and Kevin Teoh, *The Occupational Health Psychologist* 14 (June 2017), https://www.researchgate.net/publication/322744610_An_interview_with_Christina_Maslach.

23 "Burn-out an 'occupational phenomenon': International Classification of Diseases," World Health Organization, May 28, 2019, https://www.who.int/news/item/28–05-2019-burn-out-an-occupational-phenomenon-international-classification-of-diseases.

24 Christina Maslach and Michael Leiter, *The Burnout Challenge: Managing People's Relationships with Their Jobs* (Cambridge: Harvard University Press, 2022), 1–7.

25 Charles Figley, "Introduction: Treating Compassion Fatigue," in *Treating Compassion Fatigue*, ed. Charles Figley (New York: Brunner-Routledge, 2002), 2.

26 Charles Figley, "Compassion Fatigue: Toward a New Understanding of the Costs of Caring," in *Secondary Traumatic Stress: Self-Care Issues for Clinicians, Researchers, and Educators*, 2nd ed., ed. B. Hundall Stamm (Baltimore: Sidran Press, 1999), 10.

27 Emily Peters, "Compassion fatigue in nursing: A concept analysis," *Nursing Forum* 53, no. 4 (October/December 2018): 466–80, https://doi.org/10.1111/nuf.12274.

28 Trisha Dowling, "Compassion does not fatigue!" *Canadian Veterinary Journal* 59, no. 7 (July 2018): 749–50, PMID: 30026620.

29 Ibid.

30 Stephen Trzeciak and Anthony Mazzarelli, *Compassionomics: The Revolutionary Scientific Evidence that Caring Makes a Difference* (Pensacola, FL: Studer Group, 2019), xiv.

31 Ibid., viii–ix.

32 Ibid., 322.

33 For instance, a study by Chaiyachati et al. found that first-year interns doing inpatient internal medicine only spend 13% of their time interacting with patients, while 43% of their time is spent with the EMR. Krisda H. Chaiyachati et al., "Assessment of Inpatient Time Allocation Among First-Year Internal Medicine Residents Using Time-Motion Observations," *JAMA Internal Medicine* 179, no. 6 (June 1, 2019): 760–67, https://doi.org/10.1001/jamainternmed.2019.0095.

Another study, by Overhage and McCallie, found that each outpatient physician visit requires 16 minutes of physician time on the EMR. J. Marc Overhage and David McCallie Jr., "Physician Time Spent Using the Electronic Health Record During Outpatient Encounters: A Descriptive Study," *Annals of Internal Medicine* 172, no. 3 (February 4, 2020): 169, https://doi.org/10.7326/M18-3684.

34 Kopacz, *Re-humanizing*, 39–43, 300–12.

35 David Kopacz and Gary Orr, "The gift of burnout: initiation into becoming a healer," poster presented at Australasian Doctors' Health Conference (November 2019), Perth, Australia, https://beingfullyhuman.com/2020/01/24/the-gift-of-burnout-initiation-into-becoming-a-healer/.

36 David Kopacz, "Burnout: Soul Loss & Soul Recovery in Mental Health Care," Being Fully Human blog, March 26, 2020, https://beingfullyhuman.com/2020/03/26/burnout-soul-loss-soul-recovery-in-mental-health-care/.

37 Arthur Kleinman, "The soul in medicine," *The Lancet* 394, no. 10199 (August 2019): 630–31, https://doi.org/10.1016/S0140-6736(19)31961-0.

38 Christina Maslach and Michael Leiter, *The Truth About Burnout: How Organizations Cause Personal Stress and What to Do About It* (San Francisco: Jossey-Bass, 1997), 17.

39 Parker J. Palmer, *The Courage to Teach: Exploring the Inner Landscape of a Teacher's Life*, 10th anniversary ed. (San Francisco: John Wiley & Sons, 2007), 197.

40 John P. Miller, *Education and the Soul: Toward a Spiritual Curriculum* (Albany: State University of New York Press, 2000), 9.

41 Thomas Moore, *The Care of the Soul: A Guide for Cultivating Depth and Sacredness in Everyday Life* (New York: Harper, 1992), xvi.

42 Thomas Moore, *Soul Therapy: The Art and Craft of Caring Conversations* (New York: HarperOne, 2021), 6, 7.

43 Frédéric Dutheil et al., "Suicide among Physicians and Health-Care Workers: A Systematic Review and Meta-Analysis," *PLOS ONE* 14, no. 12 (December 12, 2019): e0226361, https://doi.org/10.1371/journal.pone.0226361.

44 Katherine J. Gold, Thomas L. Schwenk, and Ananda Sen, "Physician Suicide in the United States: Updated Estimates from the National Violent Death Reporting System," *Psychology, Health & Medicine* 27, no. 7 (2022): 1563–75, https://doi.org/10.1080/13548506.2021.1903053.

45 Louise Andrew, "Physician Suicide," Medscape, updated Jul 13, 2022, https://emedicine.medscape.com/article/806779-overview.

46 "Dr. Lorna Breen: Sister, Daughter, Friend, Physician," Dr. Lorna Breen Heroes' Foundation, accessed July 29, 2022, https://drlornabreen.org/about-lorna/.

47 "The Dr. Lorna Breen Health Care Provider Protection Act," Dr. Lorna Breen Heroes' Foundation, accessed July 29, 2022, https://drlornabreen.org/about-the-legislation/.

48 This concept of a dying away of the ego is also found in many spiritual and mystical traditions. For instance, the Sufi concept of *fana*, that "we need to die before we die." "What needs to die," according to Ergin and Johnson, "is our belief in ourselves as separate, insular beings disconnected from each other as well as from the larger world within which we live." Nevit Ergin and Will Johnson, *The Rubais of Rumi: Insane with Love* (Rochester, VT: Inner Traditions, 2007), 11. We discuss this and related concepts of becoming a mystic and visionary in *Becoming Medicine*.

49 David Rosen, *Transforming Depression: Healing the Soul through Creativity* (York Beach, ME: Nicholas-Hays, 2002), 70.

50 Eduardo Duran, *Healing the Soul Wound: Trauma-informed Counseling for Indigenous Communities*, 2nd ed. (New York: Teachers College Press, 2019), 121.

51 Lucia Thornton, *Whole Person Caring: An Interprofessional Model for Healing and Wellness* (Indianapolis, IN: Sigma Theta Tau International, 2013), xxiii.

52 Colin West et al., "Resilience and Burnout Among Physicians and the General US Working Population," *JAMA Network Open* 3, no. 7 (2020): e209385, https://doi.org/10.1001/jamanetworkopen.2020.9385.

53 David Kopacz and Lucinda Houghton, "A New Paradigm for Growth," CLOSLER, October 18, 2022, https://closler.org/lifelong-learning-in-clinical-excellence/a-new-paradigm-for-growth.

54 Richard G. Tedeschi and Lawrence G. Calhoun, "TARGET ARTICLE: 'Posttraumatic Growth: Conceptual Foundations and Empirical Evidence,'" *Psychological Inquiry* 15, no. 1 (2004): 1–18, https://doi.org/10.1207/s15327965pli1501_01.

55 Campbell focused primarily on the masculine hero's journey. Other authors have further developed the heroine's journey, for instance Maureen Murdock's *The Heroine's Journey* and Maria Tatar's *The Heroine with 1001 Faces*.

56 Michael Meade, *Awakening the Soul: A Deep Response to a Troubled World* (Vashon, WA: Greenfire Press, 2018), 73.

57 David Kopacz and Joseph Rael, *Becoming Medicine: Pathways of Initiation into a Living Spirituality* (Seattle, WA and Marvel, CO: Condor & Eagle Press, 2020), 43–49.

58 Michael Murphy, *The Future of the Body: Explorations into the Further Evolution of Human Nature* (New York: Jeremy P. Tarcher/Putnam, 1992), 558.

59 Plotinus, *The Enneads*, abridged ed., ed. John Dillon, trans. Stephen MacKenna (New York: Penguin Books, 1991), 22. In footnote 25, page 22, Dillon points out that Plotinus is referencing "the Stoic doctrine of the mutual implication' (*antakolouthia*) of the virtues."

60 Online Etymology Dictionary, s.v. "embody," accessed January 14, 2023, http://www.etymonline.com/index.php?term=embody.

61 Stanley Keleman, *Myth & the Body: A Colloquy with Joseph Campbell* (Berkeley: Center Press, 1999), 20.

62 Shyamala Iyer, "Atoms & Life," Arizona State University School of Life Sciences Ask a Biologist, September 27, 2009, https://askabiologist.asu.edu/content/atoms-life.

63 Moore, *Care of the Soul*, xix.

64 Plato, *Charmides (Extracts)*, trans. Benjamin Jowett (1892), David Jordan's UCSD website, last modified September 27, 2019, https://pages.ucsd.edu/~dkjordan/arch/greeks/PlatoCharmides.html#:~:text=For%20this%2C%E2%80%9D%20he%20said%2C,cure%2C%20without%20the%20charm.%E2%80%9D.

65 "Empedocles," *The Cambridge Dictionary of Philosophy*, 2nd ed., ed. Robert Audi (New York: Cambridge University Press, 1999), 261–2. Also see Peter Kingsley's book *Reality*.

66 *Merriam-Webster Online Dictionary*, s.v. "quintessence," accessed November, 1, 2022, https://www.merriam-webster.com/dictionary/quintessence. Also see Jung's writings on alchemy. "The light of nature is the *quinta essentia*, extracted by God himself from the four elements, and dwelling 'in our hearts,'" (citing *Astronomia magna*, ed. Sudhoff, XII, pp. 36 and 304), in C.G. Jung, *The Collected Works of C.G. Jung*, vol. 13, *Alchemical Studies*, (Princeton, NJ: Princeton University Press, 1968), 115 (¶ 148).

67 Bessel van der Kolk, *The Body Keeps the Score: Brain, Mind, and Body in the Healing of Trauma* (New York: Penguin Books, 2015), 12. Also see chapter 6, "Losing Your Body, Losing Your Self."

68 Stephen Cope, *Yoga and the Quest for the True Self* (New York: Bantam Books, 2000), 107.

69 David Kopacz and Joseph Rael, "Making America Healthy Again: Indigenous Perspectives on Land & Health," *About Place Journal*, Vol. VI, Issue III, May 2021, https://aboutplacejournal.org/issues/geographies-of-justice/ways-of-seeing/david-r-kopacz-md-and-joseph-rael-beautiful-painted-arrow/.

70 Substance Abuse and Mental Health Services Administration, *SAMHSA's Concept of Trauma and Guidance for a Trauma-Informed Approach*, HHS Publication No. (SMA) 14-4884 (Rockville, MD: Substance Abuse and Mental Health Services Administration., 2014) https://ncsacw.acf.hhs.gov/userfiles/files/SAMHSA_Trauma.pdf.

71 Online Etymology Dictionary, s.v. "animus," accessed March 25, 2022, https://www.etymonline.com/word/animus?ref=etymonline_crossreference.

72 Walt Whitman, "Song of Myself," *The Walt Whitman Reader: Selections from Leaves of Grass* (Philadelphia: Courage Books/Running Press, 1993), 53.

73 Whitman, "I Sing the Body Electric," Ibid., 119.

74 Walt Whitman, "Our Wounded and Sick Soldiers," *New York Times* December 11, 1864: 1–2, in The Walt Whitman Archive, accessed March 25, 2022, https://whitmanarchive.org/published/periodical/journalism/tei/per.00200.html.

75 Rachel Allyn, *The Pleasure Is All Yours: Reclaim Your Body's Bliss and Reignite Your Passion for Life* (Boulder: Shambhala, 2021), 2.

76 Benjamin Baddeley, Sangeetha Sornaligam, and Max Cooper, "Sitting is the new smoking: Where do we stand?" *British Journal of General Practice* 66, no. 646 (May 2016): 258, https://doi.org/10.3399/bjgp16X685009.

77 Daniel Odier, *Yoga Spandakarika: The Sacred Texts at the Origins of Tantra* (Rochester, VT: Inner Traditions, 2005), 2.

78 Lorin Roche, *The Radiance Sutras: 112 Gateways to the Yoga of Wonder & Delight* (Boulder: Sounds True, 2014), 15–17.

79 Tom Vitale, "Music Is Everywhere: John Cage At 100," All Things Considered, NPR, September 5, 2012, https://www.npr.org/2012/09/05/160618202/music-is-everywhere-john-cage-at-100.

80 Online Etymology Dictionary, s.v. "passion," accessed March 25, 2022, https://www.etymonline.com/word/passion.

81 Alan S. Waterman et al., "The Questionnaire for Eudaimonic Well-Being: Psychometric Properties, Demographic Comparisons, and Evidence of Validity," *The Journal of Positive Psychology* 5, no. 1 (2010): 41–61, https://doi.org/10.1080/17439760903435208. Also see Alan Waterman, ed., *The Best Within Us: Positive Psychology Perspectives on Eudaimonia* (Washington DC: American Psychological Association, 2013).

82 Online Etymology Dictionary, s.v. "eudaimonic," accessed October 20, 2023, https://www.etymonline.com/word/eudaemonic.

83 Richard C. Miller, *The iRest Program for Healing PTSD: A Proven-Effective Approach to Using Yoga Nidra Meditation & Deep Relaxation Techniques to Overcome Trauma* (Oakland, CA: New Harbinger Publications, 2015), 53.

84 Stephen Cope, *Yoga and the Quest for the True Self* (New York: Bantam Books, 2000), 107.

85 Rana Awdish, *In Shock: My Journey from Death to Recovery and the Redemptive Power of Hope* (New York: Picador, 2017), 239.

86 Joseph Campbell and Bill Moyers, *The Power of Myth* (New York: Anchor Books, 1991), 4–5.

87 Maslach, interview, Kinman and Teoh.

88 Esther Sternberg, *The Balance Within: The Science Connecting Health and Emotions* (New York: W.H. Freeman & Company, 2001), 15.

89 Ibid., 16.

90 C.G. Jung, *The Collected Works of C.G. Jung*, vol. 6, *Psychological Types* (Princeton, NJ: Princeton University Press, 1971). Also see *The Essential Jung: Selected and Introduced by Anthony Storr* (Princeton, NJ: Princeton University Press, 1983) for shorter excerpts of Jung's writing on psychological types and individuation.

91 Online Etymology Dictionary, s.v. "emotion," accessed January 15, 2023, http://www.etymonline.com/index.php?term=emotion&allowed_in_frame=0.

92 van der Kolk, *Body*, 101.

93 Wikipedia, s.v. "Robert Plutchik," accessed January 15, 2023, https://en.wikipedia.org/wiki/Robert_Plutchik#/media/File:Plutchik-wheel.svg.

94 "Universal Emotions," Paul Ekman Group, accessed January 15, 2023, https://www.paulekman.com/universal-emotions/.

95 I have written an essay on this topic, "Learning To Save the Self," available on my website, https://www.davidkopacz.com/published-articles/learning-to-save-the-self.

96 Samuel Shem, *The House of God* (New York: Berkley, 2010), 293.

97 Ibid., 303.

98 Ibid., 300.

99 Kopacz, *Re-humanizing*, 314–15.

100 Maslach, interview, Kinman and Teoh.

101 "They May Forget What You Said, But They Will Never Forget How You Made Them Feel," Quote Investigator, April 6, 2014, https://quoteinvestigator.com/2014/04/06/they-feel/.

102 Maslach and Leiter, *Truth*, 29–30.

103 Mukta Panda, *Resilient Threads: Weaving Joy and Meaning into Well-Being* (Palisade, CO: Creative Courage Press, 2020), 144.

104 See Leonard Wisneski and Lucy Anderson, *The Scientific Basis of Integrative Medicine*, 2nd ed. (New York: CRC Press, 2009), 96–7.

105 Yunli Zhao et al., "Living Alone and All-Cause Mortality in Community-Dwelling Adults: A Systematic Review and Meta-Analysis," *EClinicalMedicine* 54 (December 2022): 101677, https://doi.org/10.1016/j.eclinm.2022.101677.

106 Mwenya Mubanga et al., "Dog Ownership and Survival After a Major Cardiovascular Event: A Register-Based Prospective Study," *Circulation: Cardiovascular Quality and Outcomes* 12, no. 10 (2019): e005342, https://doi.org/10.1161/CIRCOUTCOMES.118.005342.

107 Dean Ornish et al., "Effect of comprehensive lifestyle changes on telomerase activity and telomere length in men with biopsy-proven low-risk prostate cancer: 5-year follow-up of a descriptive pilot study," *The Lancet Oncology* 14, no. 11 (October 2013): 1112–20, https://doi.org/10.1016/S1470–2045(13)70366–8.

108 Sternberg, *Balance Within*, 3.

109 Miller, *iRest Program for Healing PTSD*, 97.

110 Jalāl al-Dīn Rumi, "The Guest House," *The Essential Rumi: New Expanded Edition*, trans. Coleman Barks (New York: HarperOne, 2004), 10; online with permission, Scottish Poetry Library, accessed January 25, 2022, https://www.scottishpoetrylibrary.org.uk/poem/guest-house/.

111 Mihaly Csikszentmihalyi, *Flow: The Psychology of Optimal Experience* (New York: Harper & Row, 1990), 49.

112 Campbell and Moyers, *Myth*, 285.

113 Henry David Thoreau, *The Portable Thoreau*, ed. Carl Bode (New York: Penguin Books, 1984), 559.

114 Glenn Branch, "Whence Lumpers and Splitters," National Center for Science Education, December 2, 2014, https://ncse.ngo/whence-lumpers-and-splitters. Branch writes that the use of these terms pre-dated Darwin, although Darwin is often credited with originating the terms.

115 Iain McGilchrist, *The Master and His Emissary: The Divided Brain and the Making of the Western World* (New Haven, CT: Yale University Press, 2019), 174–5.

116 McGilchrist, *Master*, 171.

117 Jiddu Krishnamurti, *Total Freedom* (San Francisco: HarperSanFrancisco, 1996), 116.

118 Ibid., 29.

119 Daniel Simons and Christopher Chabris, "Gorillas in Our Midst: Sustained Inattentional Blindness for Dynamic Events," *Perception* 28, no. 9 (1999): 1059–74, https://doi.org/10.1068/p281059. The authors have a website about the experiment, http://www.theinvisiblegorilla.com/gorilla_experiment.html.

120 Trafton Drew, Melissa Võ, and Jeremy Wolfe, "The Invisible Gorilla Strikes Again: Sustained Inattentional Blindness in Expert Observers," *Psychological Science* 24, no. 9 (2013): 1848–53, https://doi.org/10.1177/0956797613479386.

121 Pema Chödrön, *The Wisdom of No Escape: And the Path of Loving-Kindness* (Boston: Shambhala Publications, 1991), 33.

122 Thoreau, *Portable*, 562–63.

123 Jon Kabat-Zinn, *Mindfulness for Beginners: Reclaiming the Present Moment—and Your Life* (Boulder: Sounds True, 2012), 1.

124 Iain McGilchrist, *The Matter With Things: Our Brains, Our Delusions, and the Unmaking of the World, Volume 2: What Then Is True?* (London: Perspectiva Press, 2021), 1214.

125 Christiane Wolf and J. Greg Serpa, *A Clinician's Guide to Teaching Mindfulness: The Comprehensive Session-by-Session Program for Mental Health Professionals and Health Care Providers* (Oakland: New Harbinger Publications, 2015), 22.

126 Christopher Germer, "Mindfulness: What Is It? What Does It Matter?" in *Mindfulness and Psychotherapy*, 2nd ed., ed. Christopher Germer, Ronald Siegel, and Paul Fulton (New York: The Guilford Press, 2013), 14.

127 *Jacob's Ladder*, directed by Adrian Lyne (Los Angeles, CA: Carolco & Tri-Star Pictures, 1990), 1 hour, 53 minutes.

128 Viktor Frankl, *Man's Search for Meaning* (Boston: Beacon Press, 2006), 112, Kindle.

129 Ibid., 66.

130 Ibid., 138.

131 François Lelord, *Hector and the Search for Happiness* (New York: Penguin Books, 2010). The list builds throughout the book, but 127–129 has a partial summary up to number 19.

132 Jon Kabat-Zinn, *Full Catastrophe Living: Using the Wisdom of Your Body and Mind to Face Stress, Pain, and Illness*, rev. ed. (New York: Bantam, 2013), xxxv.

133 Ramana Maharshi, *Be as You Are: The Teachings of Sri Ramana Maharshi*, ed. David Godman (New York: Arkana, 1985), 57.

134 Mark Epstein, *The Trauma of Everyday Life* (New York: Penguin, 2013), 87.

135 Online Etymology Dictionary, s.v. "evolve," accessed March 31, 2022, https://www.etymonline.com/word/evolve#etymonline_v_11717.

136 Online Etymology Dictionary, s.v. "evolution," accessed March 31, 2022, https://www.etymonline.com/word/evolution.

137 Ken Wilber, *A Brief History of Everything* (Boston: Shambhala, 1996), 30.

138 Ibid., 10.

139 David Bohm, *On Creativity* (New York: Routledge, 1996), 12.

140 Ibid., 97.

141 Ibid., 135.

142 Dean Ornish, *Love & Survival: 8 Pathways to Intimacy and Health* (New York: Harper Collins, 1998), 11.

143 Elisabeth Kübler-Ross, *The Wheel of Life: A Memoir of Living and Dying* (New York: Scribner, 2012), 285–6, Kindle.

144 Online Etymology Dictionary, s.v. "compassion," accessed March 31, 2022, http://www.etymonline.com/index.php?term=compassion.

145 Online Etymology Dictionary, s.v. "health," accessed March 31, 2022, https://www.etymonline.com/search?q=health..

146 Trzeciak and Mazzarelli, *Compassionomics*, vii.

147 Ibid., xv.

148 Ibid., xiv.

149 Philip K. Dick, "The Android and the Human," in *The Shifting Realities of Philip K. Dick: Selected Literary and Philosophical Writings*, ed. Lawrence Sutin, (New York: Vintage Books, 1995), 191.

150 Robin Youngson, *Time to Care: How to Love Your Patients and Your Job* (Raglan, New Zealand: RebelHeart Publishers, 2012), 165.

151 Kopacz, *Re-humanizing*, 310.

152 Awdish, *In Shock*, 244.

153 Ibid., 3.

154 Arthur Kleinman, *The Soul of Care: The Moral Education of a Husband and a Doctor* (New York: Viking, 2019), 32, 37.

155 Ibid., 4–5.

156 Ibid., 219–22.

157 Ibid., 220.

158 John P. Miller, *The Holistic Curriculum*, 3rd ed. (Toronto: University of Toronto Press, 2019), 7–17.

159 Adapted from David Kopacz and Joseph Rael, *Walking the Medicine Wheel: Healing Trauma and PTSD* (Tulsa, OK: Pointer Oak, 2016), 164–65.

160 From the American Holistic Medical Association's "Principles of Holistic Medicine," cited in Kopacz, *Re-humanizing Medicine*, 106. The American Holistic Medical Association no longer exists, having morphed into the Academy of Integrative Health & Medicine (AIHM) in 2014, which has slightly different list of "Core Values" of integrative health on their website https://aihm.org/about/. To me, there is an important distinction between "holistic" and "integrative," which I discuss in *Re-humanizing Medicine*, 97–99. Integrative medicine can be practiced as adding a select few Complementary and Integrative Medicine (CIM) evidence-based techniques into standard contemporary medical practice; For instance, prescribing herbs or supplements that have a degree of evidence-base. Holistic medicine, to me, encompasses more than evidence-based medical techniques, going beyond the mind and the intellect to include human dimensions of heart, intuition, and spirit. To put it another way, an integrative medicine practitioner might *do* different things than a standard contemporary practitioner, and yet not *be* different. Holistic medicine includes the human development of the healer in contradistinction to forms of medicine that rely on technical interventions. Holistic medicine is about heart to heart, whereas integrative medicine can be from the mind of the practitioner to the body of the patient.

161 Francis Peabody, "The Care of the Patient," *JAMA* 88, no.12 (March 19, 1927): 877–82.

162 M. Scott Peck, *The Road Less Travelled* (London: Arrow, 1978), 69.

163 Wayne Teasdale, *The Mystic Heart: Discovering a Universal Spirituality in the World's Religions* (Novato, CA: New World Library, 1999), 122.

164 Cited in Kopacz, *Re-humanizing Medicine*, 106. The American Holistic Medical Association (AHMA) existed from 1978 to 2013 and then merged into the Academy of Integrative Health & Medicine (AIHM). Thus, the original "principles of holistic medicine" are no longer available as a primary reference on the internet. I still have a copy of them as a poster on my clinic office door and I also used them as the framework for chapter 4 in *Re-humanizing Medicine*. See endnote 160.

165 Jean Watson, *Unitary Caring Science: The Philosophy ad Praxis of Nursing* (Louisville, CO: University Press of Colorado, 2018), 49.

166 Ibid., 46.

167 "The King Philosophy—Nonviolence 365," The King Center, accessed March 11, 2022, https://thekingcenter.org/about-tkc/the-king-philosophy/.

168 Martin Luther King Jr., *Strength to Love* (Boston: Beacon Press, 2019), 68–69, Kindle.

169 Gerald Arbuckle, *Humanizing Healthcare Reforms* (London: Jessica Kingsley, 2013). Refounding will be discussed in chapter 10 on leadership.

170 Gerald Arbuckle, *From Chaos to Mission: Refounding Religious Life Formation* (Homebush, NSW: St. Pauls Publications, 1996), 116.

171 Robert Moore, *The Archetype of Initiation: Sacred Space, Ritual Process, and Personal Transformation* (Bloomington, IN: Xlibris, 2001), 89, 140.

172 Kopacz and Rael, *Becoming Medicine*, 426.

173 The 14th Dalai Lama (Tenzin Gyatso), in Mark Epstein, *The Zen of Therapy: Uncovering a Hidden Kindness in Life* (New York: Penguin Press, 2023), 277.

174 C. G. Jung, *Modern Man in Search of a Soul* (New York: Harcourt, 1933), 49, 53.

175 Malynn Utzinger, "Enhancing Heart Rate Variability," in *Integrative Medicine*, ed. Rakel and Minichiello, 788.

176 See the Research Sections at HeartMath Institute's website, https://www.heartmath.org/research/, as well Wisneski and Anderson, *Scientific Basis*, 183–85.

177 Utzinger, "Enhancing," 787–95.

178 Erika Friedmann and Sue Thomas, "Pet Ownership, Social Support, and One-Year Survival after Acute Myocardial Infarction in the Cardiac Arrhythmia Suppression Trial (CAST)," *American Journal of Cardiology* 76, no. 17 (December 1995): 1213–17, https://doi.org/10.1016/S0002–9149(99)80343–9.

179 James Fowler and Nicholas Christakis, "Dynamic spread of happiness in a large social network: longitudinal analysis over 20 years in the Framingham Heart Study," *British Medical Journal* 337 (December 2008), doi: https://doi.org/10.1136/bmj.a2338.

180 Kaitlyn Petruccelli, Joshua Davis, and Tara Berman, "Adverse Childhood Experiences and Associated Health Outcomes: A Systematic Review and Meta-Analysis," *Child Abuse & Neglect* 97 (2019): 104127, https://doi.org/10.1016/j.chiabu.2019.104127.

181 Marco Iacoboni, "The Mirror Neuron Revolution: Explaining What Makes Humans Social," interview by Jonah Lehrer, *Scientific American*, July 1, 2008, https://www.scientificamerican.com/article/the-mirror-neuron-revolut/.

182 Personal communication with Michael Lee, Ceremonial Elder, American Lake VA Hospital Sweat Lodge; Blackfeet Nation; root tiospaye Thunder Elk Valley-Lakota Nation (April 17, 2023).

183 Joseph Rael, *Ceremonies of the Living Spirit* (Tulsa, OK: Council Oak Books, 1997), 101.

184 John Prendergast, "The Sacred Mirror: Being Together," in *The Sacred Mirror: Nondual Wisdom and Psychotherapy*, ed. John Prendergast, Peter Fenner, and Sheila Krystal (St. Paul, MN: Paragon House, 2003), 98.

185 Ibid., 115.

186 Kurt Vonnegut, letter to Xavier High School, November 5, 2006, republished in "Kurt Vonnegut On Making Your Soul Grow," Writers Write, accessed November 4, 2022, https://www.writerswrite.co.za/kurt-vonnegut-on-making-your-soul-grow/.

187 Donald Winnicott, "Playing: Creative Activity and the Search for the Self," in *Playing and Reality* (New York: Routledge, 1989), 54.

188 Susannah Heschel recounting the words of her father, Rabbi Heschel, cited in *Life Between the Trees* (blog), August 6, 2012, https://lifebetweenthetrees.wordpress.com/2012/08/06/words-create-worlds-monday-morning-parable/.

189 Genesis 1:3 (Revised Standard Version, Second Catholic Edition).

190 John 1:1 (RSV).

191 Lewis Mehl-Madrona, *Healing the Mind Through the Power of Story: The Promise of Narrative Psychiatry* (Rochester, VT: Bear & Company, 2010), 2.

192 Ibid., 2.

193 Ibid, 5.

194 Joseph Rael, *Sound: Native Teachings and Visionary Art* (Tulsa, OK: Council Oak Books, 2009), 11.

195 Louise DeSalvo, *Writing as a Way of Healing: How Telling Our Stories Transforms Our Lives* (New York: HarperCollins, 1999), 3.

196 Rachel Kulchar and Mira-Belle Haddad, "Preventing Burnout and Substance Use Disorder among Healthcare Professionals through Breathing Exercises, Emotion Identification, and Writing Activities," *Journal of Interprofessional Education & Practice* 29 (December 2022): 100570, https://doi.org/10.1016/j.xjep.2022.100570.

197 Gita Anjali Narayan, Penny Stern, and Alice Fornari, "Effect of Reflective Writing on Burnout in Medical Trainees," *MedEdPublish* 7 (2018): 237, https://doi.org/10.15694/mep.2018.0000237.1.

198 David Kopacz, "I stare out," *Body Electric: Journal of the Medical Humanities*, Volume IX, 1993, also on my website: https://www.davidkopacz.com/published-poetry/i-stare-out.

199 Hilton Koppe, *One Curious Doctor: A Memoir of Medicine, Migration and Mortality* (Melbourne: Hambone Publishing, 2022), 9.

200 Opening up past traumas can often bring on more symptoms, such as poor sleep, nightmares, and flashbacks. This is to be expected as you first work with trauma. If you feel overwhelmed, always seek support through crisis lines or therapists.

201 Hilton Koppe's website, accessed March 15, 2022, https://www.hiltonkoppe.com/Media.php.

202 Chris Smith, *Be a Good Story* (Milwaukee: Academy for Mindfulness, 2023).

203 "Poetry Collections," David Kopacz website, accessed March 15, 2022, https://www.davidkopacz.com/poetry.

204 Jill Bormann Mantram Repetition Program, accessed March 15, 2022, https://www.jillbormann.com/.

205 Betty Edwards, *Drawing on the Right Side of the Brain,* 4th ed. (New York: TarcherPerigree, 2012), 11.

206 Shaun McNiff, *Art Heals: How Creativity Cures the Soul* (Boulder: Shambhala, 2004), v, italics in original.

207 Ibid., 176.

208 Mimi Farrelly-Hansen, *Spirituality and Art Therapy: Living the Connection* (Philadelphia: Jessica Kingsley Publishers, 2001), 24–25.

209 McNiff, *Art Heals*, xii–xiii.

210 Ibid., 53–54.

211 Hippocrates, *Aphorismi*, 1, *The Genuine Works of Hippocrates*, trans. Charles Darwin Adams (1868), Perseus Digital Library, Tufts University, accessed March 18, 2022, https://www.perseus.tufts.edu/hopper/text?doc=Perseus%3atext%3a1999.01.0248%3atext%3dAph.

212 Julia Cameron, *The Artist's Way: A Spiritual Path to Higher Creativity* (New York: TarcherPerigee, 2016), 9.

213 Jalāl al-Dīn Rumi, "Someone Digging in the Ground," trans. Coleman Barks, in *The Soul is Here for its Own Joy: Sacred Poems from Many Cultures,* ed. Robert Bly (Hopewell, NJ: The Ecco Press, 1995), 166.

214 Rael, *Sound,* 1

215 Rael, *Ceremonies*, 90–91.

216 Joseph Rael and David Kopacz, *Becoming Who You Are: Beautiful Painted Arrow's Life & Lessons for Children Ages 10–100* (Seattle, WA and Marvel, CO: Condor & Eagle Press, 2021), 46.

217 Michael Meade, *The Genius Myth* (Vashon, WA: GreenFire Press, 2016), 15–16.

218 Ibid., 16–17.

219 Sally Atkins and Melia Snyder, *Nature-Based Expressive Arts Therapy* (Philadelphia: Jessica Kingsley Publishers, 2018), 60.

220 Ibid., 49.

221 James Hillman, *Healing Fiction* (Putnam, CT: Spring Publications, 1994), 4.

222 C. G. Jung, *Memories, Dreams, Reflections* (New York: Vintage Books, 1989), 171.

223 Jalāl al-Dīn Rumi, "In Baghdad, Dreaming of Cairo," summarized from *The Essential Rumi: New Expanded Edition*, trans. Coleman Barks (New York: HarperOne, 2004), 206–11.

224 Online Etymology Dictionary, s.v. "intuit," accessed March 31, 2022, https://www.etymonline.com/word/intuit.

225 McGilchrist, *Matter*, 706.

226 1 Kings 19:11–13 (New King James Version).

227 August Kekulé in O. Theodore Benfey, "August Kekule and the Birth of the Structural Theory of Organic Chemistry in 1858," *Journal of Chemical Education* 35, no. 1 (January 1958): 21, https://doi.org/10.1021/ed035p21.

228 This is a recounting of a dream I had in which the dog represented a shadow figure, initially frightening and later helpful. The dog was black in the dream. This could be interpreted as a racist stereotype, that what was frightening was "black," yet in the dream it was also a positive guide, so the use of "black" could have both a positive and negative connotation. Fear of the dark in humans likely preceded any kind of racial projections around pigmented skin. In working with the unconscious, blackness is often associated with the unknown and with unconsciousness itself. The night sky is black, and when you open your eyes in an underground cave, you see black, an absence of light. My description of the dog as black represents my dream experience; it is not meant to contribute to racial stereotyping.

229 Robert Johnson, *Inner Work: Using Dreams and Active Imagination for Personal Growth* (New York: HarperCollins, 1986), 51.

230 Ibid., 55.

231 Rael, *Ceremonies*, 40.

232 This is different than my understanding of the use of vision boards with which someone tries to manifest something in their lives. The visioning I am talking about is an emptying or opening of the ego so that the unconscious or the sacred can appear in images to guide the ego, rather than the ego trying to get something it wants in the world.

233 Henry Corbin, *Spiritual Body and Celestial Earth: From Mazdean Iran to Shī'te Iran* (Princeton, NJ: Princeton University Press, 1989), 177.

234 Henry Corbin, *Alone with the Alone: Creative Imagination in the Sūfism of Ibn 'Arabī* (Princeton, NJ: Princeton University Press, 1998), 3.

235 For a discussion of the relationship between Jung and Corbin, see Peter Kingsley, *Catafalque: Carl Jung and the End of Humanity* (London: Catafalque Press, 2018).

236 Corbin, *Alone*, 4.

237 Rael, *Ceremonies*, 80.

238 Ibid., 87.

239 *The Red Book: Liber Novus* is available in a hardcover edition, about 12" x 16", and it is an expensive book. The *Reader's Edition* is a standard sized book, but does not have any artwork, just the text. If you just want to see some of Jung's paintings, you can look online: "C. G. Jung's *Red Book: Liber Novus*," Philemon Foundation, https://philemonfoundation.org/published-works/red-book/.

240 C. G. Jung, *The Red Book: Liber Novus*, ed. Sonu Shamdasani (New York: W.W. Norton & Company, 2009), 232; *The Red Book: Liber Novus: A Reader's Edition* (New York: W.W. Norton & Company, 2012), 127.

241 Ibid., 233, (*Reader's Edition*, 133).

242 Jung, *Memories*, 199.

243 Online Etymology Dictionary, s.v. "receive," accessed March 11, 2022, https://www.etymonline.com/word/receive.

244 Kopacz and Rael, *Becoming Medicine*, 13.

245 Kopacz and Rael, *Becoming Medicine*, 455.

246 We write about this in Kopacz and Rael, *Medicine Wheel*, 50, 59, 131.

247 Joseph Rael, *Being & Vibration: Entering the New World* (Graham, NC: Millichap Books, 2015), 69–70. Originally with Mary Elizabeth Marlow, *Being & Vibration* (Tulsa, OK: Council Oak Books, 1993).

248 Girard writes that "pharmakon in classical Greek means both poison and the antidote for poison, both sickness and cure—in short, any substance capable of perpetrating a very good or a very bad action." René Girard, *Violence and the Sacred*, trans. Patrick Gregory (Baltimore, MD: Johns Hopkins University Press, 1979), 95.

249 Kopacz and Rael, *Becoming Medicine*, 23.

250 Thornton, *Whole Person*, 79.

251 Online Etymology Dictionary, s.v. "spirit," accessed March 11, 2022, https://www.etymonline.com/word/spirit.

252 Online Etymology Dictionary, s.v. "whole," accessed March 11, 2022, https://www.etymonline.com/word/whole.

253 David Tacey, *Gods and Diseases: Making Sense of our Physical and Mental Wellbeing* (Sydney: HarperCollins, 2011), 209.

254 Harold Koenig, "Religion, Spirituality, and Health: A Review and Update," *Advances in Mind-Body Medicine* 29, no. 3 (2015): 19–26, PMID: 26026153.

255 Online Etymology Dictionary, s.v. "chakra," accessed March 11, 2022, https://www.etymonline.com/word/chakra.

256 C. G. Jung, *The Psychology of Kundalini Yoga: Notes of the Seminar Given in 1932* (Princeton, NJ: Princeton University Press, 1996), 85, 61.

257 Pierre Teilhard de Chardin, *Hymn of the Universe*, trans. Gerald Vann (New York: Harper Colophon Books, 1969), 62.

258 Online Etymology Dictionary, s.v. "holism, accessed March 11, 2022, https://www.etymonline.com/word/holistic.

259 Vincent Di Stefano, *Holism and Complementary Medicine: Origins and Principles* (Crows Nest, NSW: Allen & Unwin, 2006), 92.

260 Teasdale, *Mystic Heart*, 5.

261 Ibid., 105–106.

262 Ibid., 437.

263 Dame Julian of Norwich, in *The Common Experience*, ed. J.M. Cohen and J-F. Phipps (Los Angeles: J.P. Tarcher, 1979), 111.

264 Teasdale, *Mystic Heart*, 53.

265 Larry Dossey, *Reinventing Medicine: Beyond Mind-Body to a New Era of Healing* (San Francisco: HarperSanFrancisco, 1999), 24.

266 Ibid., 31–32.

267 Larry Dossey, *One Mind: How Our Individual Mind Is Part of a Greater Consciousness and Why it Matters* (Carlsbad, CA: Hay House, 2014), xxi.

268 Ibid., 259.

269 Richard Miller, "Welcoming All That Is: Nonduality, Yoga Nidra, and the Play of Opposites in Psychotherapy," in *Sacred Mirror*, eds. Prendergast, Fenner, and Krystal, 227.

270 Conversation with Joseph Rael (Beautiful Painted Arrow), February 28, 2020.

271 Dan Millman, *Way of the Peaceful Warrior: A Book That Changes Lives* (Tiburon, CA: H J Kramer, Inc., 1984), 113.

272 Jack Mezirow, "Transformational Learning Theory," in *Transformative Learning in Practice: Insights from Community, Workplace, and Higher Education*, ed. Jack Mezirow, Edward Taylor, and Associates (San Francisco: Jossey-Bass, 2009), 19. Mezirow's model has ten steps; these referenced are steps one, four, and ten in Mezirow's model.

273 Ibid., 25.

274 Michael Meade, *Awakening*, 24.

275 Ibid., 72–73.

276 Ibid., 10.

277 Ibid., 120.

278 Ibid., 128.

279 Victor Turner, *The Ritual Process: Structure and Anti-Structure*, The Lewis Henry Morgan Lectures 1966 (New York: Aldine de Gruyter, 1995), 94–95. Turner expanded upon the earlier work of Arnold van Gennep's *rites de passage*. The concept of initiation was also later crucial to Joseph Campbell's development of the concept of the hero's journey. The hero's journey is another term for initiation.

280 Eduardo Duran and Bonnie Duran, *Native American Postcolonial Psychology* (Albany: State University of New York Press, 1995), 63.

281 Chuang Tzu, *Chuang Tzu: Basic Writings*, trans. Burton Watson (New York: Columbia University Press, 1964), 45.

282 Atkins and Snyder, *Nature-Based*, 35.

283 Fritjof Capra and Pier Luisi, *The Systems View of Life: A Unifying Vision* (Cambridge, UK: Cambridge University Press, 2014), xii.

284 Ibid., xi.

285 Online Etymology Dictionary, s.v. "harmony," accessed March 18, 2022, http://www.etymonline.com/index.php?allowed_in_frame=0&search=harmony&searchmode=none.

286 Wen-Tzu, *Wen-Tzu*, in *The Taoist Classics: The Collected Translations of Thomas Cleary*, vol. 1, trans. Thomas Cleary (Boston: Shambhala, 1999), 168–69.

287 Kopacz and Rael, *Becoming Medicine*, 53.

288 Esther Sternberg, *Healing Spaces: The Science of Place and Well-being* (Cambridge, MA: The Belknap Press of Harvard University Press, 2009), 1–2.

289 Roger S. Ulrich, "View Through a Window May Influence Recovery from Surgery," *Science* 224, no. 4647 (April 27, 1984): 420–21, https://doi.org/10.1126/science.6143402.

290 Sternberg, *Healing Spaces*, 220.

291 James Oschman, *Energy Medicine: The Scientific Basis* (New York: Churchill Livingstone, 2000), 108. Discussion of the Schumann resonance is found on pages 97–104, 107–110, and 183–186.

292 Edward Tick, *Soul Medicine: Healing through Dream Incubation, Visions, Oracles, and Pilgrimage* (Rochester VT: Healing Arts Press, 2023), 3.

293 Peter Kingsley, *In the Dark Places of Wisdom* (Point Reyes Station, CA: The Golden Sufi Center, 1999), 80.

294 Tony Schwartz, Jean Gomes, and Catherine McCarthy, *The Way We're Working Isn't Working* (New York: Free Press, 2010), 3.

295 Danielle Ofri, "The Business of Health Care Depends on Exploiting Doctors and Nurses," *New York Times*, June 8, 2019, https://www.nytimes.com/2019/06/08/opinion/sunday/hospitals-doctors-nurses-burnout.html.

296 Victor Montori, *Why We Revolt: A Patient Revolution for Careful and Kind Care* (St. Paul, MN: The Patient Revolution, 2017), 45, 5.

297 Maslach and Leiter, *Burnout Challenge*, 66–67.

298 Ibid., 232–33.

299 Capra and Luisi, *Systems*, xi.

300 Carol Schaefer, *Grandmothers Counsel the World: Women Elders Offer Their Vision for Our Planet* (Boston: Shambhala, 2006), 1, Kindle.

301 Rael, *Sound*, 256.

302 Andrew Lisa, "How long it takes 50 common items to decompose," Stacker, updated April 14, 2023, https://stacker.com/stories/2682/how-long-it-takes-50-common-items-decompose.

303 "A Guide to Plastics in the Ocean," National Ocean Service, accessed March 1, 2022, https://oceanservice.noaa.gov/hazards/marinedebris/plastics-in-the-ocean.html.

304 For a history of nuclear testing and activist protests see Rebecca Solnit, *Savage Dreams: A Journey into the Hidden Wars of the American West* (Oakland, CA: University of California Press, 2014).

305 Robert Jay Lifton, *The Climate Swerve: Reflections on Mind, Hope, and Survival* (New York: The New Press, 2017), xii.

306 Eric Chivian and Aaron Bernstein, eds., *Sustaining Life: How Human Health Depends on Biodiversity* (New York: Oxford University Press, 2008), xi.

307 Lukoye Atwoli et al., "Call for Emergency Action to Limit Global Temperature Increases, Restore Biodiversity, and Protect Health," *BMJ* 374 (September 5, 2021): n1734, https://doi.org/10.1136/bmj.n1734.

308 Jacqui Wise, "Climate Crisis: Over 200 Health Journals Urge World Leaders to Tackle 'Catastrophic Harm,'" *BMJ* 374 (September 5, 2021): n2177, https://doi.org/10.1136/bmj.n2177.

309 Sue Stuart Smith, *The Well-Gardened Mind: The Restorative Power of Nature* (New York: Scribner, 2020).

310 Douglas Tallamy, *Nature's Best Hope: A New Approach to Conservation That Starts in Your Yard* (Portland: Timber Press, 2019). See also the Home Grown National Park website, https://homegrownnationalpark.org/about.

311 "Native Plants Finder," Home Grown National Park, accessed March 18, 2022, https://homegrownnationalpark.org/native-plants-finder.

312 "Pollinator-Friendly Native Plant Lists," Xerces Society, accessed March 18, 2022, https://xerces.org/pollinator-conservation/pollinator-friendly-plant-lists.

313 Past Events, The Doctor as a Humanist, accessed March 18, 2022, https://doctorasahumanist.weebly.com/past-events.html.

314 David Kopacz, "Being a Naturalist to Improve the Health of All," CLOSLER, March 9, 2022, https://closler.org/lifelong-learning-in-clinical-excellence/being-a-naturalist-to-improve-the-health-of-everyone.

315 Yumiko Coffey et al., "Understanding Eco-anxiety: A Systematic Scoping Review of Current Literature and Identified Knowledge Gaps," *The Journal of Climate Change and Health* 3 (August 2021): 100047, https://doi.org/10.1016/j.joclim.2021.100047; Panu Pihkala, "Anxiety and the Ecological Crisis: An Analysis of Eco-Anxiety and Climate Anxiety," *Sustainability* 12, no. 19 (2020): 7836, https://doi.org/10.3390/su12197836.

316 Online Etymology Dictionary, s.v. "ecology," accessed March 20, 2022, https://www.etymonline.com/word/ecology.

317 "7 Things You Didn't Know About Plastic (and Recycling)," National Geographic Society Newsroom, April 4, 2018, https://blog.nationalgeographic.org/2018/04/04/7-things-you-didnt-know-about-plastic-and-recycling/#:~:text=RECYCLING%20PLASTIC%20DOWNGRADES%20ITS%20QUALITY.&text=Every%20time%20plastic%20is%20recycled,can%20no%20longer%20be%20used.

318 John De Graaf, David Wann, and Thomas H. Naylor, *Affluenza: How Overconsumption Is Killing Us—and How We Can Fight Back*, 3rd ed. (San Francisco: Berrett-Koehler Publishers, 2014).

319 Anne Case and Angus Deaton, *Deaths of Despair and the Future of Capitalism* (Princeton, NJ: Princeton University Press, 2020).

320 Sam Quinones, *Dreamland: The True Tale of America's Opiate Epidemic* (New York: Bloomsbury, 2015).

321 Richard Wilkinson and Kate Pickett, *The Spirit Level: Why Greater Equality Makes Societies Stronger* (New York: Bloomsbury, 2010), 3.

322 Donald Berwick, "The Moral Determinants of Health," *JAMA* 324, no. 3 (2020): 225–26, https://doi.org/10.1001/jama.2020.11129.

323 Resmaa Menakem, *My Grandmother's Hands: Racialized Trauma and the Pathway to Mending Our Hearts and Bodies* (Las Vegas: Central Recovery Press, 2017).

324 Rhonda Magee, *The Inner Work of Racial Justice: Healing Ourselves and Transforming Our Communities through Mindfulness* (New York: TarcherPerigee, 2019), 6.

325 Ibid., 6–7.

326 Ibid., 331–32.

327 Martin Luther King, *A Testament of Hope: The Essential Writings and Speeches of Martin Luther King, Jr*, ed. James Melvin Washington (San Francisco: HarperSanFrancisco, 1991), 18.

328 Ibid., 254.

329 Edith Turner, *Among the Healers: Stories of Spiritual and Ritual Healing around the World* (Westport CT: Praeger, 2006), 141.

330 Ibid., 159.

331 Lyanda Lynn Haupt and Helen Nicholson, illust. *Rooted: Life at the Crossroads of Science, Nature, and Spirit* (New York: Little, Brown Spark, 2021), 21.

332 Carl Von Essen, *Ecomysticism: The Profound Experience of Nature as Spiritual Guide* (Rochester, VT: Bear & Co, 2010), 111.

333 Edward O. Wilson, "Biophilia and the Conservation Ethic," in *The Biophilia Hypothesis*, reissue ed., ed. Stephen R. Kellert and Edward O. Wilson (New York: Island Press, 1995), 31.

334 Charles Foster, *Being a Beast: Adventures Across the Species Divide* (New York: Picador, 2016), 1.

335 Ibid., 9.

336 Ibid., 26.

337 Ibid., 27.

338 Barry Lopez, *Horizon* (New York: Vintage Books, 2019), 26.

339 John M. Darley and C. Daniel Batson, "'From Jerusalem to Jericho': A Study of Situational and Dispositional Variables in Helping Behavior," *Journal of Personality and Social Psychology* 27, no. 1 (1973): 100–08, https://doi.org/10.1037/h0034449.

340 Watson, *Unitary Caring Science*, 146.

341 Tarthang Tulku, *Sacred Dimensions of Time and Space* (Berkeley, CA: Dharma Publishing, 1997), xxix.

342 Heraclitus, #36, in *Fragments*, trans. Brooks Haxton (New York: Penguin Classics, 2003), 25.

343 Online Etymology Dictionary, s.v. "grow," accessed April 3, 2023, https://www.etymonline.com/word/grow.

344 Mirabai Starr, *Wild Mercy: Living the Fierce and Tender Wisdom of the Women Mystics* (Boulder, CO: Sounds True, 2019), 152.

345 Michael Meade, *Why the World Doesn't End: Tales of Renewal in Times of Loss* (Seattle: GreenFire Press, 2012), 3.

346 Ibid., 73.

347 Richard C. Miller, interview by David Kopacz, The POV, August 19, 2022, https://www.the-pov.com/richard-c-miller.

348 Meade, *Why the World Doesn't End*, 37.

349 Epstein, *Trauma of Everyday*, 42.

350 Meade, *Why the World Doesn't End*, 189.

351 Kopacz and Rael, *Becoming Medicine*, 327.

352 Dina Glouberman, *The Joy of Burnout: How the End of the World Can Be a New Beginning* (Norfolk, UK: Skyrosbooks, 2002), 11.

353 Jalāl al-Dīn Rūmī, *The Rubais of Rumi: Insane with Love*, trans. Nevit O. Ergin and Will Johnson, (Rochester, VT: Inner Traditions, 2007), 11.

354 Jaideva Singh, *Spanda-Kārikās: The Divine Creative Pulsation* (Delhi: Motilal Banarsidass Publishers, 2014), 17. *Spanda* is one of the closest principles I have found to Joseph Rael's view of existence as *being & vibration*. Singh writes of *spanda*, "In reality, nothing arises, and nothing subsides. It is only the divine *Spandaśakti* which, though free of succession, appears in different aspects as if flashing in view and as if subsiding" (xviii). Kashmiri Shaivism is sometimes called nondual Shaivism, meaning that there is no self/other, no subject/object, all is of one divine substance, all is *Śiva*, all is God. "The world and *Śiva* are not two separate entities. *Śiva* is the world from the point of view of appearance, and the world is *Śiva* from the point of view of Reality. *Śiva* is both transcendent to and immanent in the world," (33). A less technical translation of this work can be found in Daniel Odier's *Yoga Spandakarika: The Sacred Texts at the Origins of Tantra* (Rochester, VT: Inner Traditions, 2005).

355 Brené Brown, *The Gifts of Imperfection: Let Go of Who You Think You're Supposed to Be and Embrace Who You Are*, 10th anniv. ed. (Center City, MN: Hazelden Publishing, 2022), xxi.

356 Robert Frost, "The Road Not Taken," reprinted on Poetry Foundation website, accessed March 31, 2022, https://www.poetryfoundation.org/poems/44272/the-road-not-taken.

357 Rebecca Solnit, *A Field Guide to Getting Lost* (New York: Penguin, 2006), 4. This question is known as Meno's paradox and is found in Plato's *Meno*. Solnit's quote may be a paraphrase. "How will you look for it, Socrates, when you do not know at all what it is? How will you aim to search for something you do not know at all? If you should meet with it, how will you know that this is the thing that you did not know?" Plato, *Meno*, 2nd ed., trans. G.M.A Grube (Indianapolis, IN: Hackett Publishing, 2012), p. 13, Kindle.

358 Ibid., 14.

359 Online Etymology Dictionary, s.v. "become," accessed March 31, 2022, https://www.etymonline.com/word/become?ref=etymonline_crossreference.

360 James Hillman, *The Soul's Code: In Search of Character and Calling* (New York: Grand Central Publishing, 1996), 6.

361 Ibid., 39.

362 Rael and Kopacz, *Becoming Who You Are*, 3.

363 Lao Tzu, *Tao Te Ching*, in *Lamps of Fire: The Spirit of Religions*, trans. Juan Mascaró (London: Methuen, 1958), 28. Mascaró notes, "Rendered from many versions by J. Mascaró."

364 Joseph Campbell, *The Hero with a Thousand Faces*, 3rd ed. (Novato, CA: New World Library, 2008), 29.

365 Palmer, *Courage*, 197.

366 Stephen Swensen and Tait Shanafelt, *Mayo Clinic Strategies to Reduce Burnout: 12 Actions to Create the Ideal Workplace* (New York: Oxford University Press, 2020), 58–59.

367 "The Vow," Order of the Sacred Earth, accessed January 18, 2023, https://www.orderofthesacredearth.org/.

368 University of Minnesota Medical School Class of 2017, "An Oath for New Physicians," *OnBeing* (blog), December 4, 2017, https://onbeing.org/blog/an-oath-for-new-physicians/. Also see Krista Tippett, "Atul Gawande: What Matters in the End," https://onbeing.org/programs/atul-gawande-what-matters-in-the-end/.

369 Larissa Thomas, Jonathan Ripp, and Colin West, "Charter on Physician Well-Being," *JAMA* 319, no. 15 (2018): 1541–42, https://doi.org/10.1001/jama.2018.1331.

370 Mukta Panda, Kevin O'Brien, and Margaret Lo, "Oath to Self-Care and Well-Being," *The American Journal of Medicine* 133, no. 2 (February 2020): 249–252.e1, https://doi.org/10.1016/j.amjmed.2019.10.001.

371 Kopacz and Rael, *Becoming Medicine*, 27–28.

372 Thich Nhat Hanh, *Being Peace* (Berkeley: Parallax Press, 2005), 88.

373 Thich Nhat Hanh, *Zen and the Art of Saving the Planet* (New York: HarperOne, 2021), 75–76.

374 Charles Eisenstein, *The More Beautiful World Our Hearts Know is Possible* (Berkeley: North Atlantic Books, 2013), 16. See also Eisenstein's *Climate: A New Story* and *The Ascent of Humanity: Civilization and the Human Sense of Self.*

375 Ibid., 21.

376 Ibid., 87.

377 Charles Foster, *Being a Human: Adventures in Forty Thousand Years of Consciousness* (New York: Metropolitan Books, 2021), 214.

378 Marc Andrus, *Brothers in the Beloved Community: The Friendship of Thich Nhat Hanh and Martin Luther King*, Jr. (Berkeley, CA: Parallax Press, 2021), 141.

379 Henri Nouwen, in Trzeciak and Mazzarelli, *Compassionomics*, 296.

380 Trzeciak and Mazzarelli, *Compassionomics*, 294–295.

381 Ibid., xiii.

382 Stephen Trzeciak and Anthony Mazzarelli, *Wonder Drug: 7 Scientifically Proven Ways that Serving Others is the Best Medicine for Yourself* (New York: St. Martin's Essentials, 2022), 6.

383 Watson, *Unitary Caring Science*, xvii.

384 "Any Idiot Can Face a Crisis; It's This Day-To-Day Living That Wears You Out," Quote Investigator, accessed March 18, 2022, https://quoteinvestigator.com/2013/06/14/face-crisis/. This quote is often incorrectly attributed to Anton Chekov.

385 Schwartz, Gomes, and McCarthy, *Working*, 21.

386 Kopacz, *Re-humanizing Medicine*, 292–293.

387 Leslie Kane, "'I Cry but No One Cares': Physician Burnout & Depression Report 2023," slide 6, Medscape, January 27, 2023, https://www.medscape.com/slideshow/2023-lifestyle-burnout-6016058#6.

388 Kopacz, *Re-humanizing Medicine*, 217.

389 Michelle Barton et al., "Stop Framing Wellness Programs Around Self-Care," *Harvard Business Review*, April 4, 2022, https://hbr.org/2022/04/stop-framing-wellness-programs-around-self-care.

390 Ibid.

391 Swensen and Shanafelt, *Strategies to Reduce Burnout*, 37.

392 Kopacz, "Beyond Resilience."

393 Online Etymology Dictionary, s.v. "resilience," accessed April 7, 2022, https://www.etymonline.com/word/resilience.

394 Edith Shiro, *The Unexpected Gift of Trauma: The Path to Posttraumatic Growth* (New York: Harvest, 2023), 60–61.

395 Tedeschi and Calhoun, "Posttraumatic Growth," 2.

396 Ibid., 4.

397 Alessandra Pigni, *The Idealist's Survival Kit: 75 Simple Ways to Avoid Burnout* (Berkeley, CA: Parallax Press, 2016), 55.

398 Swensen and Shanafelt, *Strategies to Reduce Burnout*, 281.

399 Ibid., 3.

400 Tait Shanafelt and John Noseworthy, "Executive Leadership and Physician Well-Being," *Mayo Clinic Proceedings* 92, no. 1 (January 2017): 129–46, https://doi.org/10.1016/j.mayocp.2016.10.004.

401 Pigni, *Idealist's Survival Kit*, 112.

402 Shem, *House of God*, 133.

403 Simon Talbot and Wendy Dean, "Physicians aren't 'burning out.' They're suffering from moral injury," *STAT*, July 26, 2018, https://www.statnews.com/2018/07/26/physicians-not-burning-out-they-are-suffering-moral-injury/.

404 Zubin Damania, "Stop Saying Burnout, It's Moral Injury," ZDogg MD, March 8, 2019, https://zdoggmd.com/moral-injury/.

405 William E. Flanary (@Dr. Glaucomflecken), "Wellness Exercises," Twitter, June 19, 2021, https://twitter.com/DGlaucomflecken/status/1406286232947085315?lang=en, and "The Cure for Burnout," Dr. Glaucomflecken, April 12, 2022, YouTube video, 2:39, https://www.youtube.com/watch?v=Oi8fnQjo90E.

406 William E. Flanary, "A Message On Burnout, Featuring Dr. Vivek Murthy," Dr. Glaucomflecken, December 4, 2021, YouTube video, 1:48, https://www.youtube.com/watch?v=C5tgNPOdKGM.

407 Sonya Norman and Shira Maguen, "Moral Injury," National Center for PTSD, accessed March 13, 2021, https://www.ptsd.va.gov/professional/treat/cooccurring/moral_injury.asp.

408 Patricia Watson et al., "Moral Injury in Health Care Workers," National Center for PTSD, accessed March 13, 2021, https://www.ptsd.va.gov/professional/treat/cooccurring/moral_injury_hcw.asp.

409 Wendy Dean, Simon Talbot, and Austin Dean, "Reframing Clinician Distress: Moral Injury Not Burnout," *Federal Practitioner* 36, no. 9 (September 2019): 400–02, erratum in: *Federal Practitioner* 36, no. 10 (October 2019): 447.

410 Rushton, *Moral Resilience,* there is a diagram of this schematic on page 54.

411 Ibid., 4.

412 Ibid., 13.

413 Ibid., 236.

414 Ibid., 7.

415 Ibid., 271.

416 Palmer, *Courage*, 202.

417 Ibid., 207.

418 Robert Jay Lifton, "Interview with Robert Jay Lifton," interview by David Kopacz, The POV, May 28, 2021, https://www.the-pov.com/robert-jay-lifton.

419 John Launer, "Medical Activism," *Postgraduate Medical Journal* 97, no. 1151 (September 2021): 611–12, https://doi.org/10.1136/postgradmedj-2021-140809.

420 David Kopacz, "Medical Activism: A Foundation of Professionalism," CLOSLER, December 28, 2020, https://closler.org/passion-in-the-medical-profession/medical-activism-a-foundation-of-professionalism.

421 Bandy Lee, *Profile of a Nation: Trump's Mind, America's Soul* (New York: World Mental Health Coalition, 2020), 19.

422 David Kopacz, "Words Create Worlds," 1–9, *Being Fully Human* (blog), https://beingfullyhuman.com/?s=words+create+worlds&submit=Search.

423 Susannah Heschel, cited in the *Life Between the Trees* (blog), August 6, 2012, https://lifebetweenthetrees.wordpress.com/2012/08/06/words-create-worlds-monday-morning-parable/.

424 Carl Bell, *The Sanity of Survival: Reflections on Community Mental Health and Wellness* (Chicago: Third World Press, 2004), 466. For more about the late Carl Bell, see my blog post and review of his book, "Racism & Narcissism: The Work of Carl Bell, MD," July 21, 2020, https://beingfullyhuman.com/2020/07/21/racism-narcissism-the-work-of-carl-bell-md/.

425 Paul Farmer, "General Anesthesia for the (Young Doctor's) Soul?" in *To Repair the World: Paul Farmer Speaks to the Next Generation*, ed. Jonathan Weigel (Oakland: University of California Press, 2019), 19.

426 Arbuckle, *Chaos,* 3–5.

427 Arbuckle, *Humanizing,* 70.

428 Excerpts from a 2018 email exchange between the author and Gerald Arbuckle, in Kopacz and Rael, *Becoming Medicine*, 408–410. Chapter 15 in the book is on the topic of refounding.

429 Barbara Bokhour et al., "Whole Health System of Care Evaluation–A Progress Report on Outcomes of the WHS Pilot at 18 Flagship Sites," Veterans Health Administration, Center for Evaluating Patient-Centered Care in VA (EPCC-VA), February 18, 2020, https://www.va.gov/WHOLEHEALTH/docs/EPCC-Whole-Health-System-Evaluation_2020-01-27_FINAL.pdf.

430 Alex Krist, Jeannette South-Paul, and Marc Meisnere, eds., *Achieving Whole Health: A New Approach for Veterans and the Nation*, Consensus Report of the National Academies of Sciences, Engineering, and Medicine (Washington DC: National Academies Press, 2023), 16, https://doi.org/10.17226/26854.

431 Farmer, "General Anesthesia," 5.

432 Rachel Naomi Remen interview in Krista Tippett, *Becoming Wise: An Inquiry into the Mystery and Art of Living* (New York: Penguin Books, 2016), 24–25. Permission granted.

433 Palmer, *Courage to Teach*, 206.

434 Michele Harper, *The Beauty in the Breaking* (New York: Riverhead Books, 2020), 279.

435 David Kopacz, "Yoga is Good Medicine," CLOSLER, October 6, 2020, https://closler.org/lifelong-learning-in-clinical-excellence/yoga-is-good-medicine.

436 Online Etymology Dictionary, s.v. "yoga," accessed April 29, 2023, https://www.etymonline.com/word/yoga.

437 Mark Nepo, *The Endless Practice: Becoming Who You Were Born to Be* (New York: Atria, 2014), 8–9.

438 Stephen Cope, *The Wisdom of Yoga: A Seeker's Guide to Extraordinary Living* (New York: Bantam Books, 2007), 13. Cope's discussion of *samvega* starts from its use in Patanjali's *Yoga Sutras* (1.21 – 1.22).

439 Ibid., 15.

440 Glouberman, *Joy of Burnout*, 10.

441 Ibid., 204.

442 Online Etymology Dictionary, s.v. "mentor," accessed February 25, 2023, https://www.etymonline.com/word/mentor.

443 Kopacz and Rael, *Medicine Wheel*, chapter 14 is entitled "Return to the Held-Back Place of Goodness," 251–67.

444 Arthur W. Frank, *The Wounded Storyteller: Body, Illness, and Ethics*, 2nd ed. (Chicago: University of Chicago Press, 2013), 120.

445 Ibid., 122.

446 Ibid., 123, 126.

447 Online Etymology Dictionary, s.v. "patient," accessed October 31, 2022, https://www.etymonline.com/word/patient.

448 Steven Wang, *Beating Melanoma: A Five-Step Survival Guide* (Baltimore, MD: Johns Hopkins University Press, 2011), xiii. Note that this is an older text and doesn't include the latest survival rates and treatment options of immunotherapy.

449 Frank, *Wounded Storyteller*, 71, 164.

450 Personal communication, 2022. Sam was my iRest teacher certification mentor.

451 VA Whole Health website, https://www.va.gov/wholehealth/.

INDEX

ABOUT THE AUTHOR

DAVID R. KOPACZ, MD, works as a psychiatrist in primary care at the Seattle VA and has a national position teaching Whole Health to VA staff. He is an assistant professor at the University of Washington and is board certified in psychiatry, integrative, and holistic medicine. David has spoken around the world on self-care and well-being for veterans, staff, and health professional students. He is the author of *Re-humanizing Medicine* and a number of books for adults and children with co-author Joseph Rael (Beautiful Painted Arrow), including *Becoming Medicine: Pathways of Initiation into a Living Spirituality*. Art, photography, poetry, iRest meditation and yoga, and time in nature are vital to his own well-being. Visit DavidKopacz.com.

ABOUT CREATIVE COURAGE PRESS

CREATIVE COURAGE PRESS is a small, independent publishing company founded in 2020 by Shelly L. Francis, inspired by the people she met while writing *The Courage Way: Leading and Living with Integrity* (Berrett-Koehler, 2018). Now, in collaboration with other authors, we are creating courage for the complexity of being human.

Get to know the essential voices of our remarkable authors and their refreshing ideas for leading change from the heart. Together we hope to generate meaningful conversations in our communities.

Visit us online to get fortified with resources and reflections for creating your own courageous way of life. As we grow, we invite you to grow with us.

www.CreativeCouragePress.com
hello@CreativeCouragePress.com

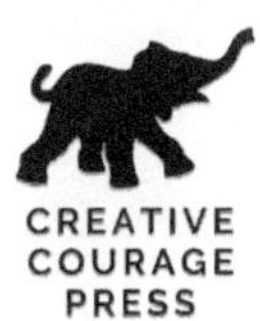

CREATIVE
COURAGE
PRESS

www.ingramcontent.com/pod-product-compliance
Lightning Source LLC
Chambersburg PA
CBHW020914060726
47591CB00004B/1241

* 9 7 8 1 9 5 9 9 2 1 0 2 8 *